SYSTEMA VOICES

Volume One

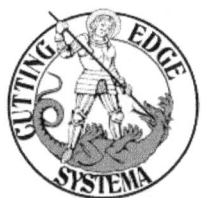

Copyright@ 2018 R Poyton

All rights reserved.

The moral right of the author has been asserted.

No part of this book may be reproduced in any form or by any electronic or mechanical means including information storage and retrieval systems, without permission in writing from the author. The only exception is by a reviewer, who may quote short excerpts in a review.

The author and publisher take no responsibility for any illness or injury resulting from practicing the exercises described in this book. Always consult your Doctor prior to training or if you have any medical issues.

Published by Cutting Edge

www.systemafilms.com

ISBN: 978-1-78926-871-3

"If you want to build a ship, don't drum up people together to collect wood and don't assign them tasks and work, but rather teach them to long for the endless immensity of the sea."

— Antoine de Saint-Exupéry

CONTENTS

SYSTEMA HQ
Daniel Ryabko 13
Larissa Ryabko 23
Vladimir Vasiliev 27
Valerie Vasiliev 33
Valentin Vasiliev 37

BRAZIL
Nelson Wagner 45

CANADA
Emmanuel Manolakakis 59
Jason Priest 73
Pete Rogers 87

CHINA
Ali Chui 105

GERMANY
Norbert Tannert 117

JAPAN
Ryo Onishi 127

PERU
Bratzo Barrena 133

TAHITI
Jerome Laigret 143

UK
Matt Hill 153
Robert Poyton 173

USA
Sergey Makarenko 193
Glen Murphy 203
Martin Wheeler 219

FOREWORD

The Russian art of Systema was unknown outside of that country up until the 1990s. Some Russian martial arts were known, the British Sombo Federation was formed in 1986, for example. Vague reports of Russian military arts also occasionally surfaced. I remember reading an article in Terry O'Neill's *Fighting Arts International* magazine for one, featuring a Spetsnaz unit practicing Karate type work with some added gymnastics and elements of Sombo.

To the best of my knowledge, the first time Systema was seen outside of Russia was when Vladimir Vasiliev moved to Toronto in the early 90s. Prior to that, information about the art is difficult to come by, due largely, perhaps, to the fact that modern Systema, as we know it, has intricate and often deep roots.

We can speculate over the post-Revolution amalgamation of family and Cossack styles; we have some knowledge about the activities of proto-Spetsnaz and counter-intelligence groups that served in both World Wars. We also have documented information on Hesychasm and other practices from the Eastern Orthodox Church as well as many writings and stories of the warriors of old.

What is clear, is that from humble beginnings Systema has now spread around the globe, to the extent that there are currently hundreds of schools and thousands of students worldwide. Workshops by Systema masters Ryabko and Vasiliev continue to draw big crowds and a large group of senior instructors also actively teach all over the world.

This is an even more remarkable fact when you consider that it was achieved with none of the trappings of "traditional" martial arts, not to mention the radically different approach of Systema. Ability speaks for itself, however, and none who have spent time with Ryabko or Vasiliev can doubt their skill and mastery, not just in the area of combat but also in the wider and deeper aspects of training. Their success has paved the way for other schools to emerge from Russia, as well producing numerous off-shoots and derivations from the original style.

It would also be fair to say that Systema's influence has reached beyond the martial arts world into areas of breath work, natural movement, health practices and more. Often unacknowledged, that influence nonetheless continues to grow.

I thought that the 25th anniversary year of the founding of the Toronto school would be an interesting time to take a "snapshot" of where Systema is right now. To that end, I've interviewed a number of Systema teachers, what you might call the first and second generation of Instructors. They range in background from special forces personnel to finance managers, musicians, LEOs, professional martial artists and more. Each has their own tale to tell and each their own view on this remarkable art, while at the same time sharing a set of core experiences. This collection also highlights the truly global nature of Systema, with contributors ranging from North and South America to Asia to Tahiti to Europe. There are some notable omissions of course; it was not possible in the time available to interview everyone that I wanted to, but I hope to include those I missed this time in Volume Two!

The interviews vary in length, which is largely down to the interview method for each person. I was fortunate to get to speak to many of the contributors in person at the *Summit of Masters* workshop in Bonn in the summer of 2018. For that, I would like to warmly thank Norbert Tannert and his team for all their help and support. Other interviews were conducted over Skype or by e-mail.

I'd also like to thank all those who kindly agreed to be interviewed and hope that the experience wasn't too harrowing! Some of these interviews were previously published in *Systema International* online magazine, though they have been revised and updated for this book. I've tried to keep editing to a minimum, I hope what comes across is the genuine voice of each Instructor. As is often the case in Systema, one question leads to another and there are many avenues left unexplored and further questions that could be asked... but we only have so much time and space!

So thank you, again, to all those who have helped in the production of this book, particularly my wife, Lara. I'd also like to thank the Ryabko and Vasiliev families, through whose tireless efforts and enthusiasm this wonderful art has been so widely shared.

Robert Poyton
Bedfordshsire, UK
October 2018

SYSTEMA HQ

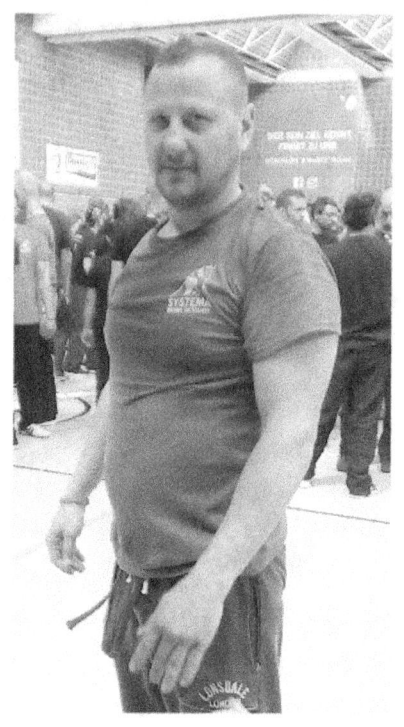

DANIEL RYABKO

Can you first tell us something about your background?

I was born in Russia, in the city of Tver, which is near Moscow. My mother was from there, also Vladimir Vasiliev, of course. Now I live in Moscow, I grew up and went to school in Moscow.

When did you first become aware of Systema?

Well there is footage of me as a toddler running round in my father's gym, so in that way I've been aware of it my whole life! But I was not so interested in it when I was a kid. At school I trained with friends and we did different martial arts, wrestling and other styles. I liked the moving around but didn't so much like having to stay in one place and do one-two, one-two type movements.

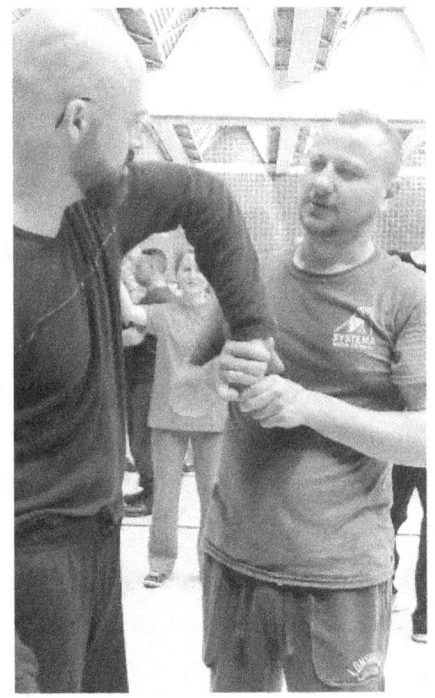

Maybe those styles need that but with Systema mentality we work in a different way.

When I first went training with my father there were other students there, I would joke with them and have fun. Then one day, I was around 13, I began to understand the great things the students were doing, so I decided to focus and begin training seriously.

I guess it was like in a movie, when I first saw martial arts. There were people training like you see in the films, I thought "Wow!". But after training with my father in Systema, I saw those same guys unable to do anything to him. Not

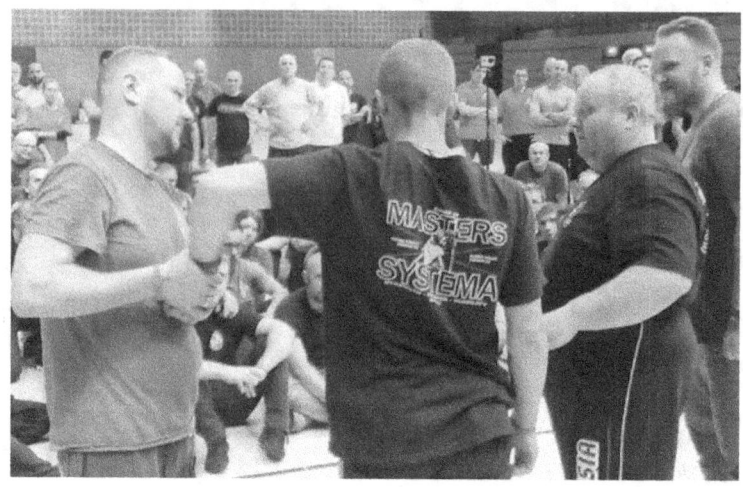

in an aggressive way but that made it clear to me that you have sports and you have martial arts, you know?

Because martial arts in movies are very showy?

Yes, and Systema is not visible in many ways. When I was a Detective in the Moscow Police there were people I worked with who were interested in sports and martial arts. Some of them were boxers, high level. They watched some of the videos I had of my father and said they couldn't understand what this stuff was, why was this guy able to do these things? Was it because they were his students? So I told them, okay, you can come to class tonight and train with us. Many did, they came to test Mikhail, some are now Instructors with us. But before, they were "what is this stuff?"

Which is natural if people don't understand what they are seeing?

Yes and at that time I said to them they could also try on me before meeting my father (laughs). It was good because they felt a different spirit from what they were used to in their own styles. Also, after I struck them they were interested to come training with Mikhail.

Do you think that this is one of the main differences between Systema and other art, the mindset, the spirit?

I think so. We are not saying bad things about other sports and styles.

Because people enjoy what they do, they like their training. It may be that if they knew something different, then they would try something else. I was at one seminar with Mikhail in Amsterdam, my friend came along to watch. He's a businessman, he's not a martial art guy at all, he'd not seen any martial arts. He saw what we did, then he asked me to go with him to look at some other gyms. He made a comment that how they trained, everything was very fast and aggressive. He suggested that perhaps that had something more to do with fear. It's an important spirit in any martial art that you don't teach people this kind of aggression. You shouldn't use fear to teach them, you know, scary faces and all that.

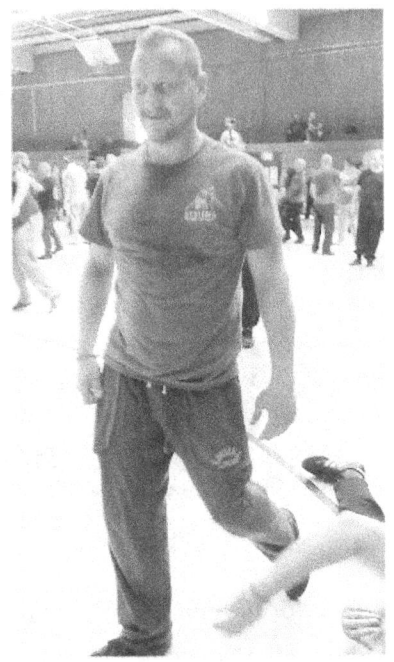

I was in Cologne with that friend, we were walking through a car park, down some steps. There was this guy at the bottom of the steps, lots of tattoos, mean face, scary looking guy. I said to my friend that this man adopts this look this for safety, right? He looks scary so people leave him alone. I smiled at the guy, he relaxed, we had a chat.

And this is a universal thing, right, how we deal with these fears?

Yes. Look around the world, wherever people are. Most of us have a family, we love mum, we love pop, you know? We love our kids. This is the same all over the world. But when you are young you are thinking about how to show yourself, how to be strong. In some countries that may be having a gun, or a knife, or to look big, have big muscles. This can be the mentality, but it is based on fear. There are some differences of course, some places are very strict on time, for example, other places are more laid back, "don't worry, soon!" you know (laughs). But we cannot say this or that is good or bad, it's just different. Aside from that, we all want the same things, to care for our families.

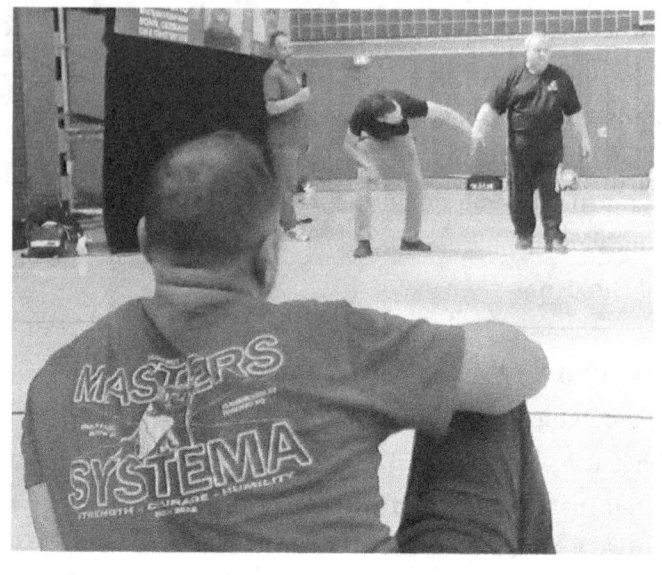

In that sense do you think that Systema training is universal?

Systema is for everyone. Some sports or martial arts are not for everyone. For example, see this elderly lady here? Let's say she goes to an MMA class, will that work out for her? Maybe, maybe not. Systema is about people, not learning to be an animal, but being people. Whoever you are, whatever age, you can benefit.

Do you think that Systema is suitable for children, too?

Yes, we have children starting from a very young age, they train with their parents. This is very good for two to five year olds, it's a great bonding experience for parents and kids. After the age of five the children generally come on their own. They learn through play.

Is this approach one of the reasons that Systema has spread so quickly around the world?

Yes. Because no-one says "this level, that level," everyone comes and trains together, all equal. In some places they make competition between people. This sometimes helps and sometimes not. For example, one guy came training. He'd seen a video and was very keen. Then after one week, he didn't come, another week, still not there. So I called him and said "you were so keen, why are you not here?" He told me he was going to the gym first to train up because he felt so bad at our school, he felt he couldn't keep up with the other students.

He thought he needed to improve before coming to us. I told him no, it is okay to come however you are. You can't do a push-up? No problem, someone will help you.

Systema is for life, it is to survive, not to prove something. We have health techniques, relaxation techniques. Even a high level sports person or boxer, they need to know how to relax.

When did you first start teaching and how did you find it?

Teaching is a big thing, yes? Because people look at you like you are the *Teacher*. What you say to them is important. So we have people teaching who have learnt from Mikhail and Vladimir. Then some of those move away, you know, they say they are doing their own "better" Systema now. Then people who train with us may invite one of those teachers to do a workshop for them.

That's okay, I have no problem with that. But the problem comes if people are not honest. I don't want that people are lied to. If you don't respect your teacher, people will never respect you. If people want to go, then fine, we say go. But there is no need to have this "best" thing going on.

Is there a difference between fighting and teaching?

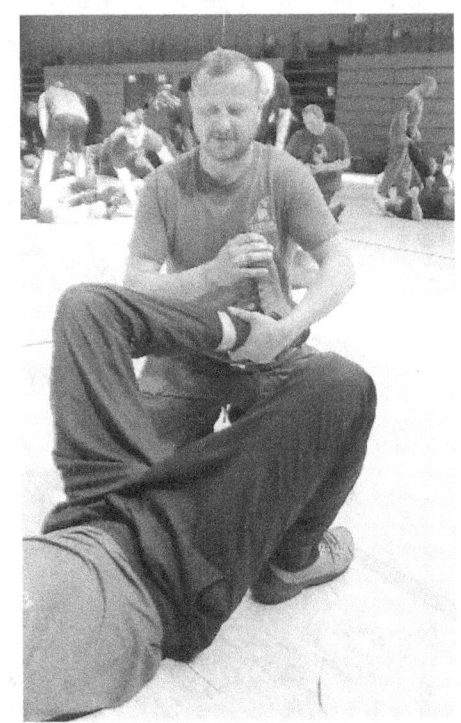

Fighters have teachers, right? Sometimes people go to the fighter and find maybe he is not such a good teacher. Teaching and fighting are two different things. A fighter can break you down. But a teacher needs to explain what they are doing, how they are doing it, how you can do it. This is why you study at university to become a teacher! In martial arts, you don't attend a few seminars and suddenly become a world-class teacher, yet this is what some people expect. They can use the name Systema, but it is more than a name. God gives knowledge to some people. One may know but not another. But I see people on the internet teaching what we were teaching ten years ago and saying it is something new. And this is why Mikhail and Vladimir gave certificates for one year only at first. Later on, once you know people, it's different.

That is why I talk about spirit. Two things give knowledge, bad things and God. So you see here today, everyone is relaxed, no animal faces, no one wants to break you. But you know how easy it is to break people, we can fall over and break ourselves! A friend of mine, sports guy, fell down some steps and broke his shoulder. I told him this is why we learn to fall and roll!

Do you think that having previous martial arts experience helps when it comes to learning Systema?

It varies from person to person. Some people come to class and try to show what they can already do, so they don't really learn what Systema is trying to teach them. Other people with experience open themselves to the training and find many things that are interesting. These things then help improve their existing skills. For example, many high-level Aikido people have come to train with us and found that their previous experience helps them learn Systema, but also that Systema helps to improve their Aikido.

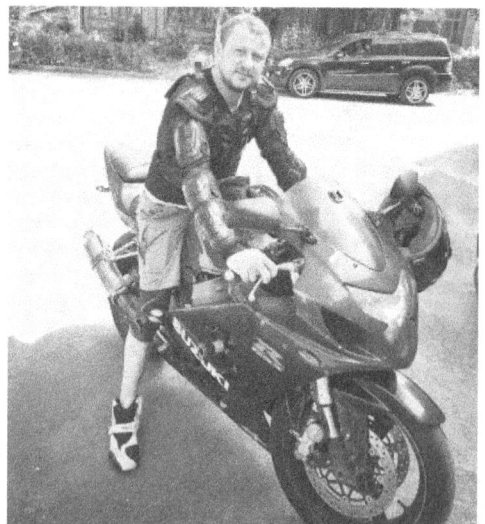

Would it be true to say that modern Systema is largely from a military background?

It is, but military work is not always how people imagine it is. For example, in the Russian military it was found that people who were overly aggressive or over emotional did not make good soldiers. A large part of Systema is learning to understand yourself and control your emotions. This helps a person to remain calm in any situation and so be able to be more effective. You can be professional in all situations. In the military sense it allows people to perform the task they need to perform. People who rely on aggression to get through everything have, I think, never been though Special Forces training.

Did you find Systema useful in your time in the police?

Yes. I was first in the police, then later Special Forces, working in counter-terrorism. I've also taught a lot of police and security in different countries. We like to teach good people, not just teach how to break people for the sake of it. Today it seems we are almost going back to Roman times, you know. Bread and gladiators. A gladiator mentality is to kill or be killed, for the entertainment of the crowd. Our way is to be peaceful, to spend time with family, Systema is for everyone. Sure, fighting if we need to, to protect. But there is more.

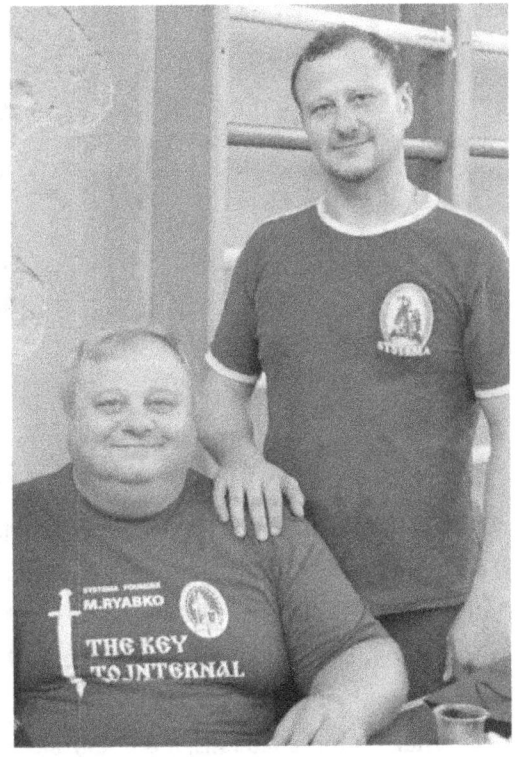

Even now in Moscow we have one of the top MMA teams coming to us. We have some banja (sauna) techniques and other things, they come, they like. Sure, for fighting their work is very specific but they are interested in how Systema makes them feel better. The body cannot lie (laughs).

And one thing that Systema does is help you listen to your body!

Yes! This is important, because when we are children we are open. Later, people say "don't do this, don't do that." So I learned some interesting things

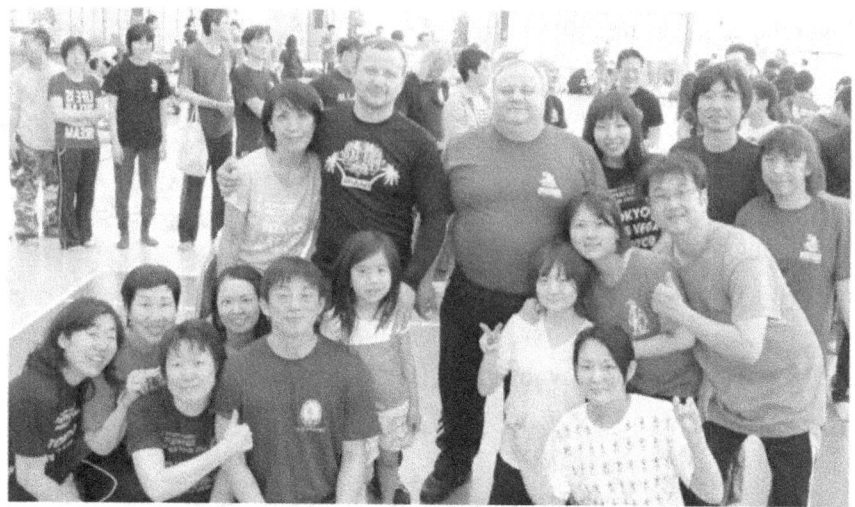

when I became a father. The first year, the baby doesn't understand so much. The next year they begin to understand things. So you say "Where is momma? Point to papa." We teach to show, to point, good boy! Then I found the year after that we say "Don't point, it's rude!". This is an interesting thing, we teach something, then say that it's bad!

When a small child falls, it is not afraid but the parents are. The child learns the fear. Of course you have to say some things, like don't put your finger in the plug socket. But you should explain why this is, because it is dangerous, you can get hurt. The explanation is very important, the kid needs to understand why. In Systema it is important we are not lazy to move, right? So also we should not be lazy to explain. People can give advice and the other person follows it and gets hurt. Then the advisor says "it was your fault." No, they should have explained the thing. Then people can understand what they are doing and if it is safe to do it.

In Russia you know, there is a saying. If someone says to you "Go there, do this, do that" then the reply is, "Okay, I go and do it, but after you" (laughs). It's a different story, then. So you have to understand why you are doing things. Are you going to the gym or a restaurant? Imagine going to the gym, setting up a table, some candles...

So it is important to get the right balance between explanation and experience?

Yes, first off people have to know what they are doing. It's important that what you know and what you do match up. People will see if it doesn't.

Systema was virtually unknown not that long ago. Now it seems that there are so many schools, in Russia and outside, teaching "Systema". Are there different styles of Systema?

Well some are now using the name Systema as a brand for their own thing. I've found that people see that, try it, then come to us and say "wow, that other stuff wasn't like this." There is a different flavour, a different spirit. Mikhail says he is the founder of Systema. Nobody knew this word before. A lot of people studied with Mikhail in the past, a lot came and tried him. Some went off but in terms of learning, they stay in the same place, they don't develop. Others try to copy.

But to move like Mikhail or Vladimir you need to be Mikhail or Vladimir! We have to understand that (laughs). We do the same, me, you. You have your way of moving, I have mine, you know, Systema is how you express yourself. Day by day that can be different. If you ask Mikhail what is similar between our school and others, he will say "nothing." It's just different people, some are good, some not too bad. For me, the most important thing is not how people train or their level but what is their personality? Bad people don't stay long in Systema. Systema protects itself.

You travel all around the world now, do you have a favourite place to visit?

I like Japan very much but everywhere else too! In each of the different countries you find something good. I think it's not the place that makes the people but the people that make the place.

Thanks for the interview and do you have any final words for the reader?

Yes - come to Systema and train!

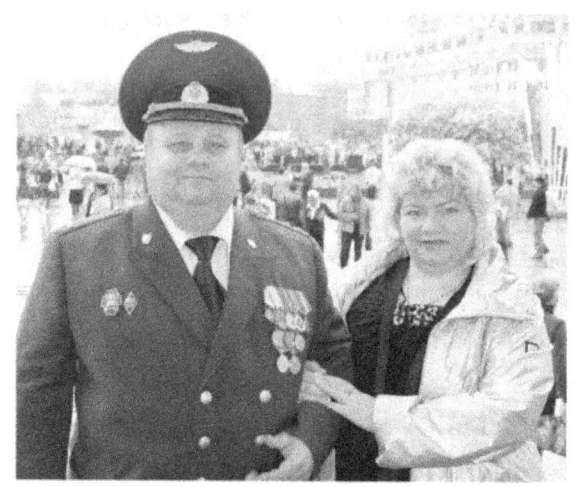

LARISSA RYABKO

Where did you first meet Mikhail and also when did you first see Systema?

This was back many years ago, Vladimir Vasiliev and I worked for the same company. There was an organised tour for the employess from the city of Tver to go to Talin. So we were on the same trip together and Mikhail joined Vladimir's group and Vladimir introduced Mikhail to me. This is our connecting link with Vladimir (laughs). When we returned home Mikhail and I began seeing each other and ended up becoming married. Before we got married Mikhail used to go diligently three times week to training class. One of the conditions of our relationship was that I would never interfere with this arrangement (laughs). So at that time I didn't really pay much attention to Mikhail's training. I knew he was doing some form of athletic activity but didn't know what it was.

Systema at that time was called "Understand Yourself". Later I became interested in where he was going so regularly, so I visited a class. I really liked it and I began training too. I trained for some time, not direct from Mikhail but from his student, for some reason I liked that better (laughs). Systema is life itself, we live it. It helps us physically and spiritually to develop and grow

Could you tell us something about the early days of teaching

Mikhail was doing his army service in Tver and after he had completed it he stayed there, working for the police. Since the time

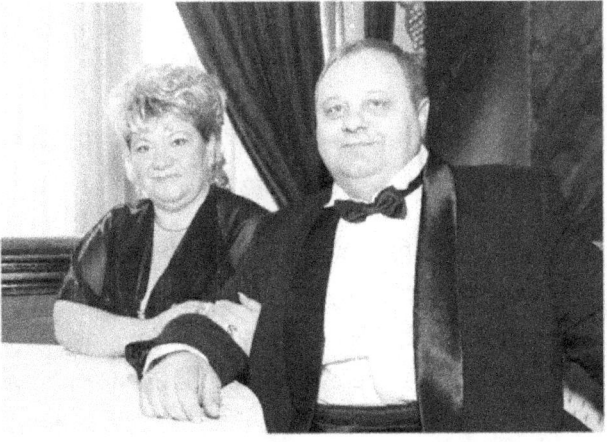

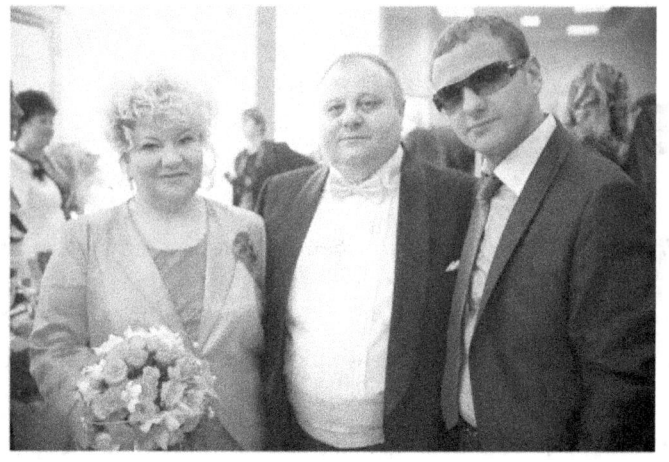

he started doing regular classes in Tver there were also many other martial arts schools there too. Vladimir who was doing all kinds of martial arts at the time, he also began Systema. So they all trained together. Many people who are well known now, I remember how they moved into Systema and stopped doing their boxing, Karate, etc.

In those years Mikhail also trained the local police and the bodyguard units in Tver. In 1989 Mikhail was transferred to work in Moscow where he started to train the bodyguards of the minister and various special forces / Spetsnaz personnel. Then of course in 1992 the government system in Russia changed dramatically.

Vladimir moved to Canada and opened his own school in Toronto in 1993. In 1999 he brought the first group of Systema students over to Moscow. Since that time the doors have been opened to Systema for the whole wide world

And now people from all the world come to visit?

Yes, I think it's over 50 countries now where people practice Systema, maybe a hundred thousand people that we know of.

It must be nice to travel and meet people, what is the favourite place and are there any you would like to see?

The great thing is that at every place we go to we see everyone has been united by Systema, so every place we visit is like home. Even though I don't know the language very well, all these people are so kind and warm, you can exchange a smile and everyone feels comfortable and happy. I've seen it time and time again, Systema protects itself. The aggressive and negative people try

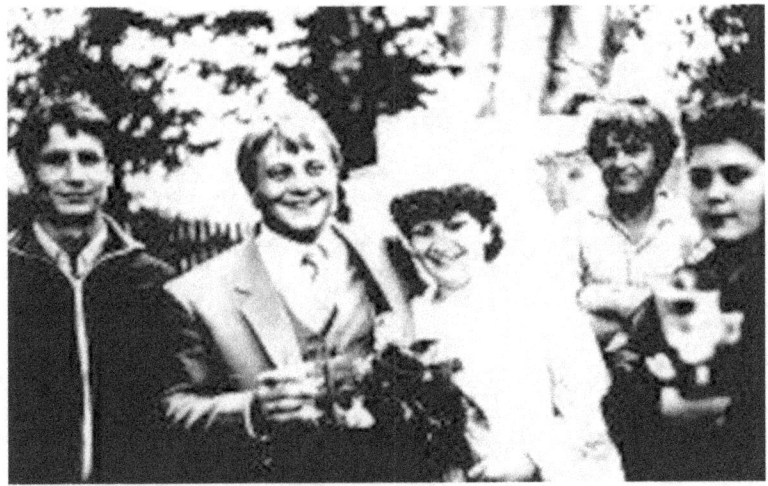

Systema for a bit, and then inevitably leave it.

I liked all the places we travelled to, Europe, Japan.... We were in Tuscany a couple of years back but never got to see Venice, I would like to visit there!

Is it good for children to learn Systema?

It is very important that kids are allowed to maintain the natural abilities they are born with. These are very easy to lose in today's technological world. Because it emphasises natural movement, Systema allows the child to maintain this natural state and thus stay healthy throughout life. The child will learn to control their body, to become strong. We have many kids in our school who train in professional sports such as tennis, skating, swimming.

They do Systema in addition to get the foundation of breathing, strength, resilience; it works very well for them in their other activities. We show them exercises to develop the muscles, ligaments particular to their kind of sport – and of course for self defence purposes too. Every person should have that, the ability to go through life without being scared.

We have a group of women too learning Systema for self defence. We could talk forever about Systema, it's such a big subject!

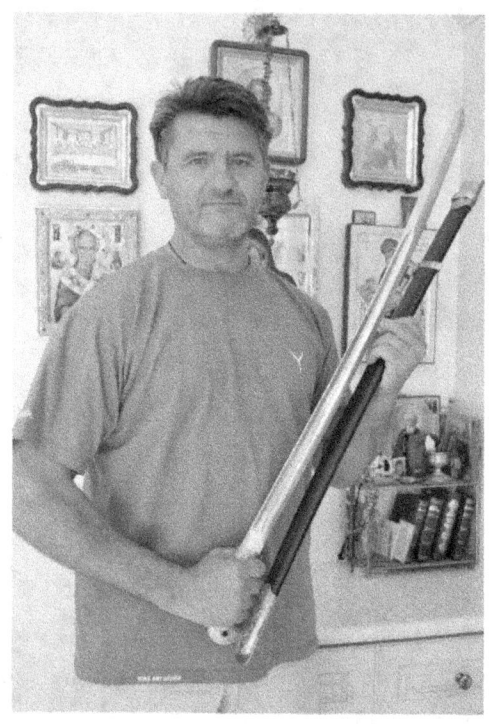

VLADIMIR VASILIEV

First of all can I say congratulations on behalf of everyone here on the 25th anniversary of your school, it's an amazing achievement! Did you have any idea when you first started teaching in Toronto that you would be in this position, with schools worldwide?

Thank you for your kind words and support. When I started teaching in Toronto in 1993, I had no plans to create something particular. Life takes its course. There are currently over 200 schools and over 700 instructors that teach Systema around the world, over 40 instructional films, regular seminars and camps with big numbers of participants. Of course, I try to put in honest work but have no set goals, I also do not depend on these developments.

You obviously trained in a lot of different things with a lot of different people in the past. What is it that drew you to Mikhail and that now makes him your source of training?

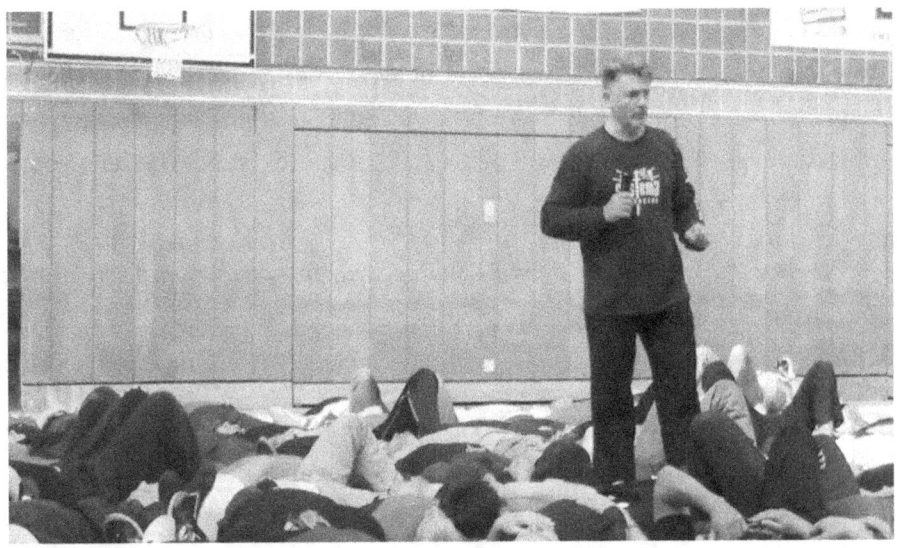

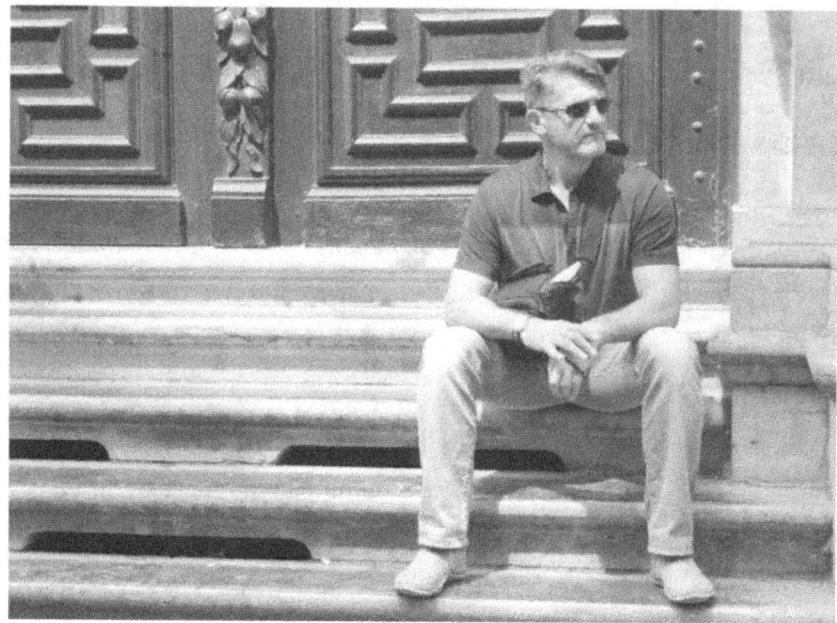

What Mikhail does is always interesting and there is always more to learn. I really like that. Seeing his top level of mastery helps me to continue working on myself.

Systema has grown incredibly over the last 25 years, do you have any thoughts as to how it might develop over the next 25 years?

I believe there is God's will for everything. I have no predictions for such distant future. I enjoy what we have today – great people and accomplishments. What I can say is that Systema is indeed unique and has a very positive effect on the practitioners. It will be great if people continue to benefit from it for the next 25 years and more.

Is there a danger that as people splinter away from the central school that the flavour changes?

There is nothing wrong if people "splinter away". We do not call for people to join, nor do we hold anyone back from leaving. It is good to explore other options. A lot of people return. Usually the ones that do not need Systema move away, they do not understand it. It is hard to comprehend and take in the whole Systema. Many people take bits and pieces of this style and think they have Systema, this is when it falls apart.

We have seen some military styles become very popular over the last few years, with a very different approach from Systema. Do you think people are surprised by Systema's military background, given its focus on health and breathing?

A good warrior is a healthy warrior, healthy in his spirit and body. Systema makes people stronger physically and also better, kinder, less fearful and less aggressive. A good warrior that is not fearful or aggressive will do a far superior job defending his country.

A lot of Systema work seems to go against the usual martial arts methods. For instance, you can punch without putting body movement in, you counter tension with relaxation and you look at yourself more than looking at the opponent. How do you best get these ideas across to people from other styles?

Practitioners need to recognize the close interaction between the health and the martial art components. Many martial arts mislead their students. In my opinion, what they teach has no relevance to health or survival. Traditionally martial arts had the goal of preservation of their generations, this is now lost.

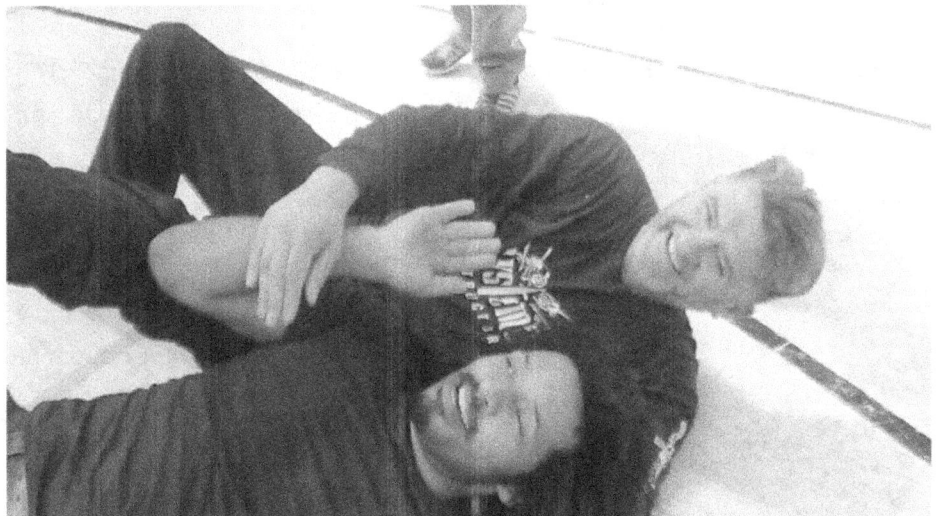

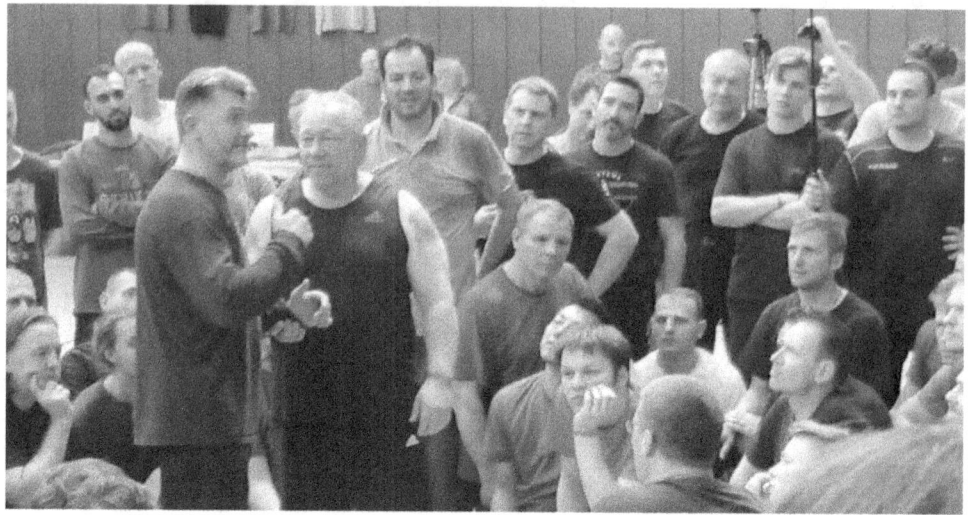

Systema's solid and natural approach and breathwork foundation brings back the right way to train, fight and live. The way a person can understand this is just by practicing himself.

People see and comment on how your own level has steadily improved over the years. How do you keep improving and what are your goals in training?

Thank you for these nice words. My goals are to gain deeper understanding of the Systema concepts. Systema is alive, it continues to develop, and this process does not end until we die. There are many examples of Systema instructors who's skill keeps growing steadily.

How do you balance being challenged and safety in training? How do you judge how much a person can take?

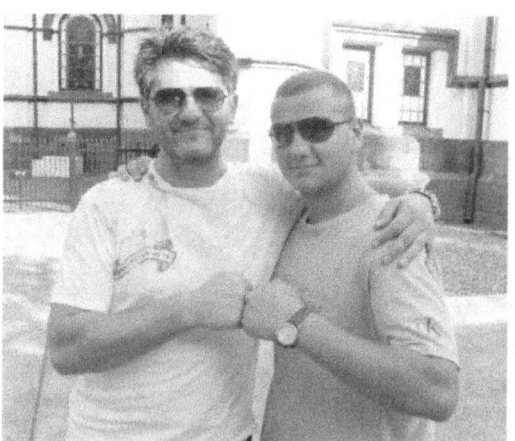

This is a great and very relevant question. This is a real challenge. If you punch hard or apply a decisive action to the opponent – he and others complain. If you do not act decisively – they do not believe you. It is testing for any instructor, especially because in Systema we work on the move. It is easy to show a convincing technique while fixed and stationary, while it is a real skill to deliver just the right dosage on the move and see to what extent your partner will let you work. As for judging how much the person can take, this is easier and comes with practice.

Do you have any stories you could share of your time training in the army, or with Mikhail?

This is a whole story in itself, perhaps we can address it sometime in the future.

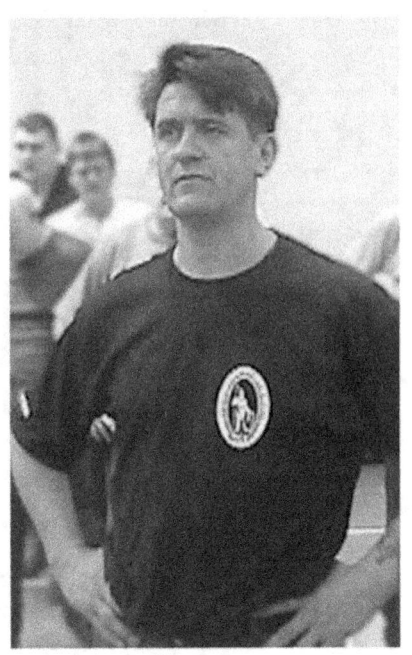

Could you give some words of advice to people new to Systema and to those who have been training for a few years?

My advice to all practitioners is to have patience. Learning Systema is an extensive process, there are challenges and rewards every step of the way. It is very exciting because new discoveries await you all the time and the profound joy of following the right path is always there.

Despite all our technology - or perhaps because of it! - there seems to be just as much uncertainty and bad events in the world as ever. Do you think Systema has a role in helping people in difficult or "interesting" times?

I am sure that it can and will help. Systema has so many applications if it is studied as a whole and not by fragments as we discussed before. Systema training reduces stress and fear, provides health and clear thinking. It really can be the source of strength and peace.

To quote Psalm 23: "Even though I walk through the valley of the shadow of death, I fear no evil, for You are with me; Your rod and Your staff, they comfort me."

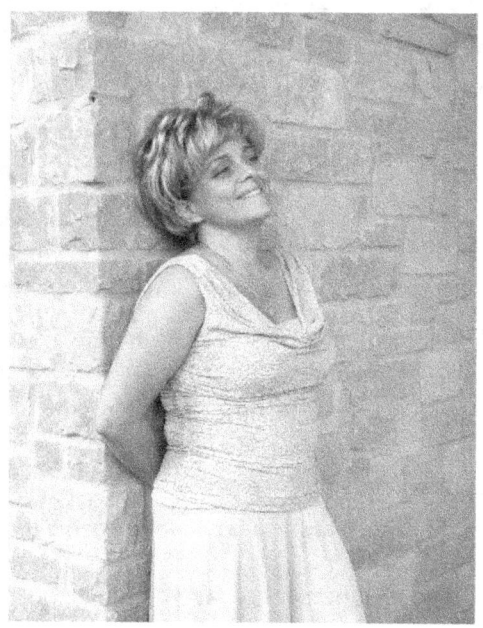

VALERIE VASILIEV

Could you please first tell us something about your background?

I was born in Russia and my family emigrated to Canada when I was a teenager. I went to school in Toronto, then later to University. There I studied psychology and physiotherapy. I became a certified physiotherapist and started working in that field. Then I met Vladimir and we got married, after that we started the school.

How did the school first begin?

Vladimir was training a small group at the local community centre to begin with. Not that he wanted to train them but people kept asking him! The group started getting bigger and bigger, until it was time to do something about it – so we started the school! That was 25 years ago and we started with twelve students, steady students. We knew they would sign up and that meant we had just enough to cover the rent and other expenses, so away we went!

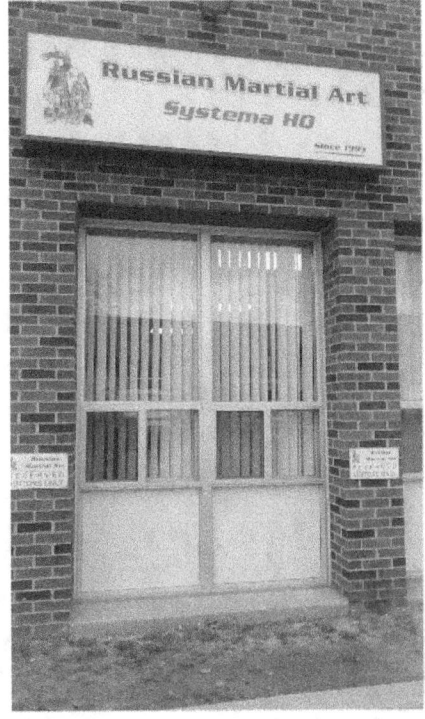

And that was at the old Glen Cameron unit?

Yes, that's right. And now, round the world we have thousands of students. There are over 700 Instructors, each with a group. Different size groups, but, yes thousands of are people now training.

That's quite an achievement and the

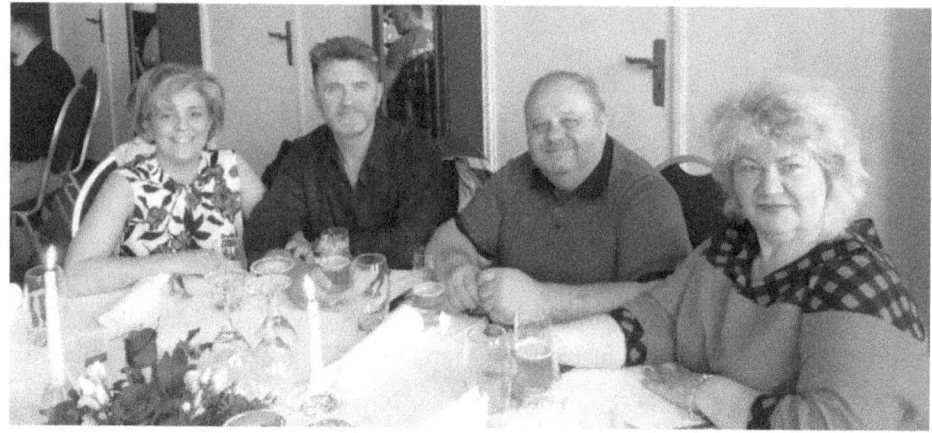

interesting thing is you have done that outside of the conventional "martial arts" way. There are no grades or buying into a franchise, for example. Did you plan it that way?

No, we never planned it as a business, or a financial thing or anything like that. It was just that Vladimir was good at teaching and many people wanted to train with him, so we started the school. As we opened the gym I was expecting our first child! Then a year later, the second child, so we were really busy! I was also doing my physiotherapy work in-between running the business and a young family. It was really difficult. Also because I never liked to use babysitters while the children were at such a young age.

How did you keep a balance between work and family life?

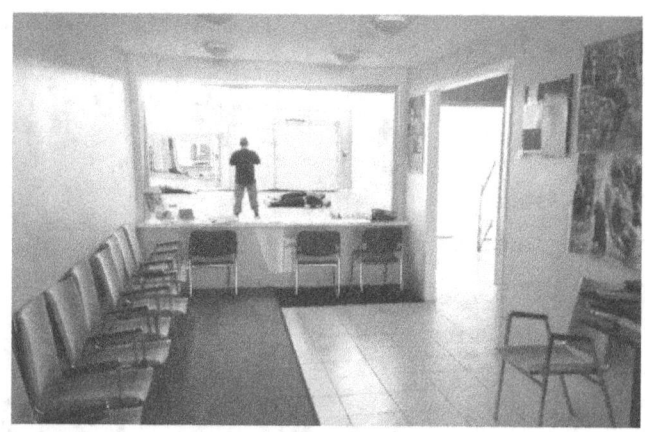

When you work together it's not so bad. Also, I believe it's God's work, as many things happened without us planning them. They just happened, somehow a lot of people appeared

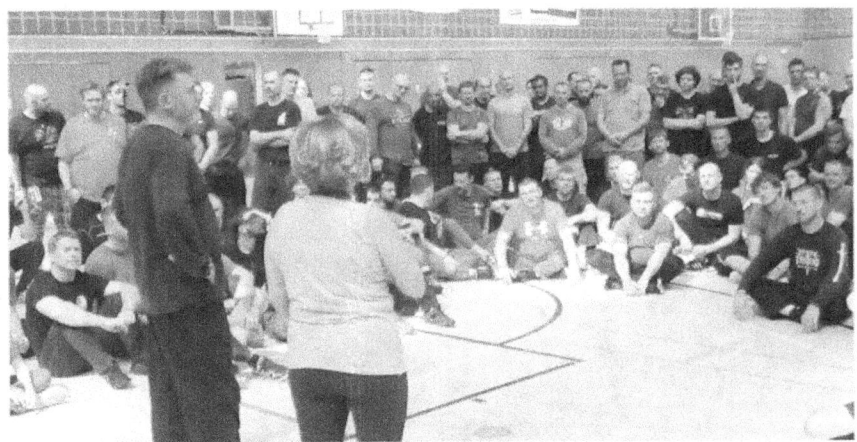

who helped us. You know, a student would come in and donate money to us. Another person would come in and install the mirrors in the gym for free, others would help with the painting and so on. So people were very helpful

Do you think that may be because Systema attracts positive people?

I think so. Systema attracts good people. That's why we had the two introductory classes before a person signed up to the school. It meant that the aggressive ones, the proud ones, they didn't stay. Those two classes were enough to put those people off.

It strikes me that the lack of aggression is one of the defining qualities of Systema?

You're absolutely right. There are many schools based on real-world combat methods but Systema differs from those schools fundamentally. Our approach says that in order to become a true warrior, you must first relax and become a stable person. Most martial arts are founded on tension and aggression. While their pupils might win a fight, they pay the price of broken bodies and traumatized psyche. Systema takes a different path, its goals are defence and healing. Though it's also worth noting that there is often a fine line between defence and attack, for instance, when you need to protect a friend or apprehend a criminal.

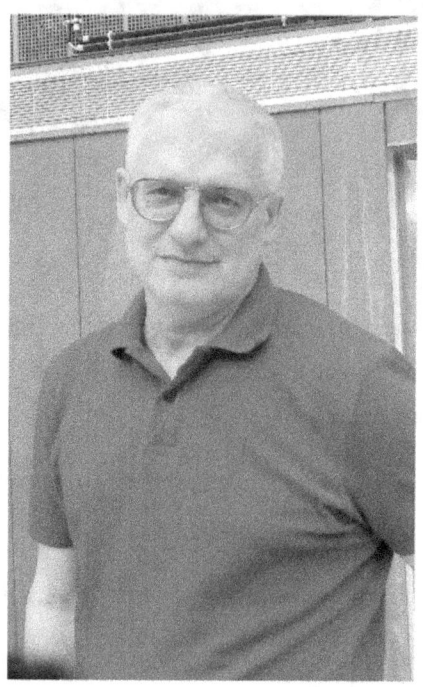

VALENTIN VASILIEV

Could we start with how you got into martial arts?

I always liked sports, such as running and swimming. I started training in martial arts for fitness and to gain confidence. I began training with Karate. I did quite well, I got first prize fighting in the Latvian Championship in Riga. At that time I knew nothing about Systema. My brother Vladimir found out about Systema first, then introduced me to it. I was always interested in something new and Systema had many things I had not seen before. Karate has a lot of rules and they don't necessarily apply to real life. I was always looking for something that applied to real life and Systema has that.

Was that something that helped in your professional life?

Very much so. Systema gave a lot more possibilities for work. But it helped with my art too. I also paint and I found it helped with creativity and expression.

We were talking about age a little bit earlier, do you find that Systema is something you can improve in with age?

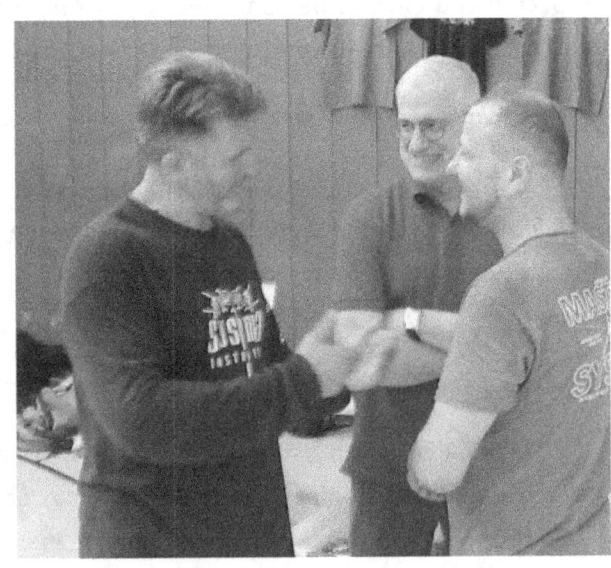

Systema becomes extremely valuable as you age. Because when you are young, you can compensate with force and power. As you get older, Systema is a real gem. You have less energy, so this is a perfect way to move without expending too

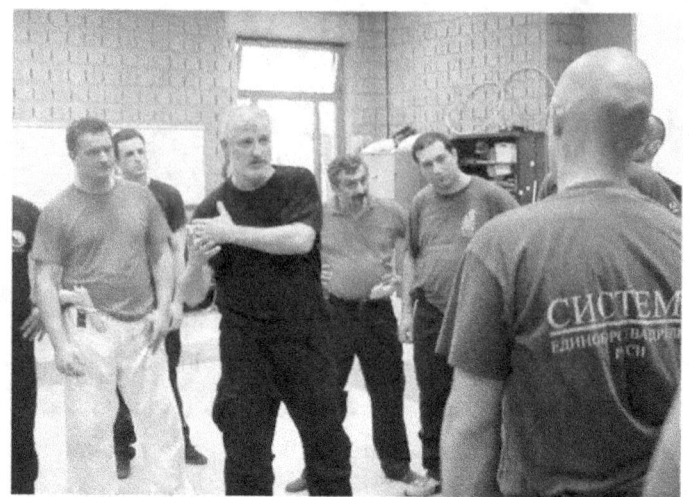

much energy.

When did you start teaching?

I first began teaching some police and special groups in Latvia - not as a professional instructor but as an amateur, people would ask me. That was teaching more SWAT type work, rather than Systema as such. But when we started training work against weapons, Systema was more effective. Because with weapons, there is no room for show. You have to improvise, to be very adaptable, Systema was perfect for that.

Also with weapons you have to be very firm, because the attacker has to be completely suppressed. Ideally the bad guy should have a real fear of authority, so there is no resistance. I feel this is what can be missing in the West, the forces don't intimidate the criminals so much. In order to be feared and respected you have to be confident in yourself, which is why you need real techniques, things that work.

Especially against weapons?

Yes. You might be a great boxer or Karate fighter, until the villain takes out a knife. In Systema the work is universal, the type of attack doesn't matter. There's no grades in Systema, yet the experience accumulates and when you need it, it will work.

Do you feel the same applies for civilian training?

I think for civilians, Systema is perfect the way it is. For professionals you have to add a little harshness. People have to be decisive if you are training for survival. Some professionals have to dominate in order to win. When violence becomes more widespread, police officers may have to become more intimidating in order to prevent violence flaring up. Police should be like a hurricane, enter, destroy everything, then back out again (laughs).

Is there a problem with the other side of that? Such as the incidents where we see of poor use of force?

Yes, in some places they use excessive force because of their weakness. They are not as professional as they should be. When arresting someone, once they are down you don't need to keep hitting them. You restrain and pick them up. The best way is when it is not clear what has happened to both the violent person and to any onlookers. The job is just done.

That brings us back to the Systema calm approach?

Yes. Because confidence comes from experience, which especially includes the breath work. Gaining experiences is a layered experience. Like a computer game! You manage one level, then you go to the next and begin again, until you become a master like Mikhail or Vladimir.

Does it help, then to have specific goals in training?

It's not necessary for a regular person but it is important for a professional. They have to set a high standard for themselves. Imagine a surgeon, they have to do their work without fear taking control. They gain that through strong experience.

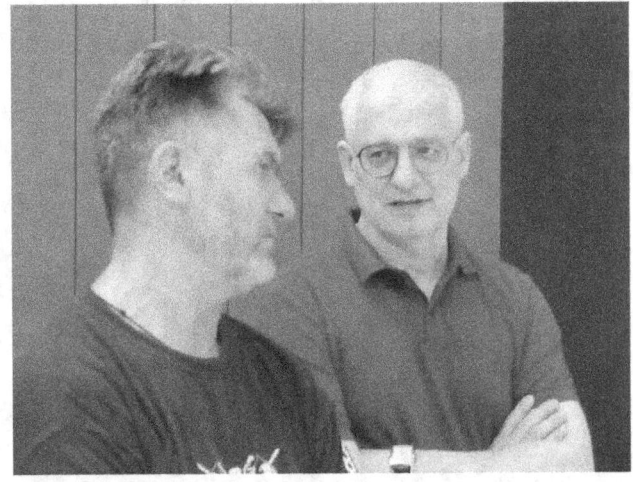

Do you think that approach also help in terms of dealing with the long term stress of being involved in that kind of work?

Yes and that is also based on experience. Because for the experienced professional, nothing is a surprise, nothing is unexpected. You see that in a situation, this or that might happen, so it doesn't stress you out. It's not planting potatoes, it's protecting people, you expect that difficult things will happen. If you look at bodyguard work, for example, that is constant awareness. As soon as you relax, something may happen.

So does that awareness become part of you, is it always there?

It's like you are walking through a jungle. You always expect there may be a snake or something around. But with experience you learn where the snakes live, which ones are poisonous, how to react to them. The same with bodyguard work, you know how many cars have been stolen that day, what to look for, where to look and so on. That constant level of adrenaline is part of the job.

Do you think that the Systema approach is good preparation for that environment?

Absolutely, yes. Because the body needs to be prepared. Sometimes people ask why are the masters showing things so slowly? They doubt that this will work in reality but this is a good method of training. If you prepare the body in this way, when it comes to use, you can move very fast, the body reacts automatically. Training this way allows the body to absorb knowledge and energy, when you need it, it is there. But it's important to check this every once in a while. For example, have two or three people attack you in class. That is

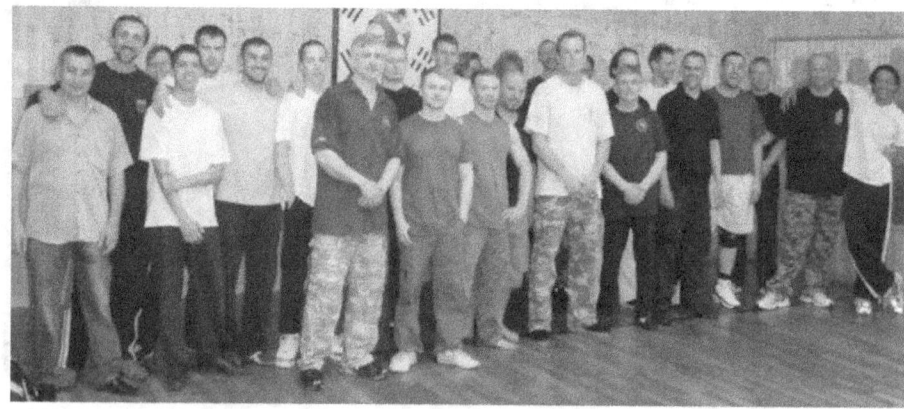

already more realistic and trains the body.

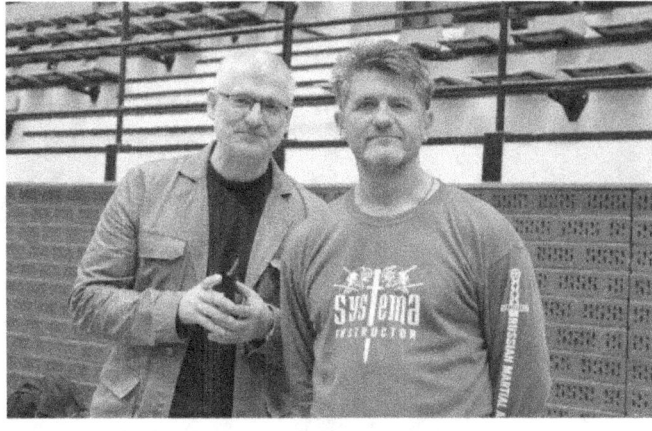

So you can to some extent test yourself in training?

Yes, it is important to test your strikes, for example. You may think that you are going to knock someone out but do you really have that ability? You have to have confidence and power in your strike, otherwise it's not a real weapon. Don't get deluded!

How do you maintain a balance between safety and testing, particularly for civilians?

First make sure that the people involved are able to deal with strikes. Second, bring your work to a conclusion. Don't just throw the person down, control them all the way through. You have to be responsible and have full control. The same will then apply in a fight. Also remember you can suppress your opponent physically or psychologically.

Do you have any advice for people in their training?

Develop real confidence and don't stop, keep working! Unusual moves have to become very usual for the body. This is where slow work really helps. Set high goals for yourself. Create challenges, have two partners attack, have one with a knife and so on. That's how you build yourself, by learning to cope with the unexpected. At the start, just work evasion, move away from the attack. But make sure it is a good attack. Have your partner throw strikes towards you, you can be standing, sitting or on the ground. Learn to move to avoid the attack, this is all good work to prepare the body.

BRAZIL

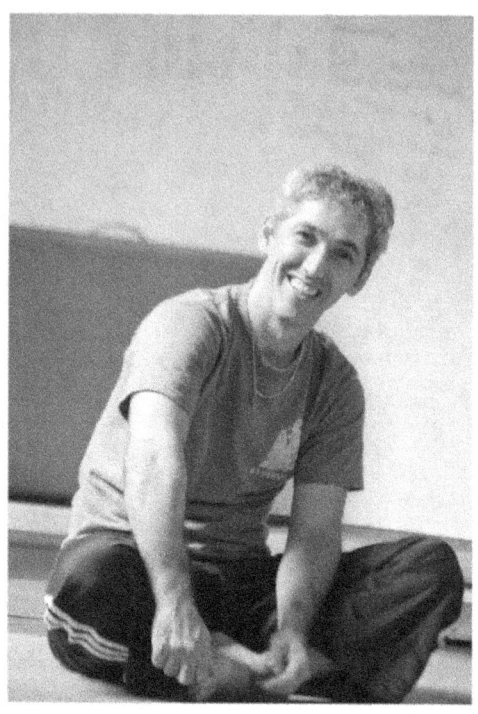

NELSON WAGNER

Could we start with something about your background?

I'm a Brazilian, born in Santos, a beach city at the coast in the state of São Paulo. I've lived most of my life in Santos and now I'm living in the city of São Paulo. My mom was a nurse and my dad was a cook, we lived in the poor areas and things were tough. I had to learn how to defend myself from bigger and older boys and men, from a small age. Back then there was a fight between boys from different neighbourhoods and, since I had to move a lot, I ended having friends and also some enemies from one place to another. Shortly after my brother was born, my parents divorced. My mom had a bad time in finding some decent partners and I had to fight in the streets and in my home. So I've looked for martial arts as a way to defend myself as I was normally the smallest one. And also got some comfort in books and learning new things.

So martial arts have always been a passion for you?

Yes. I've worked in a lot of different areas, in a bank as cashier, as a technician for an oil company, in a coffee shop roasting coffee, for example but it was through martial art that I found my passion for teaching. In 1991 I brought Aikido to Santos and started my own school, while still working in different jobs. I met an instructor of Ninjutsu and, although I

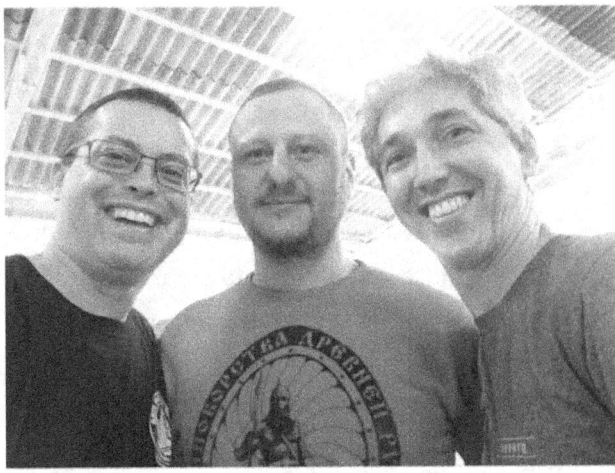

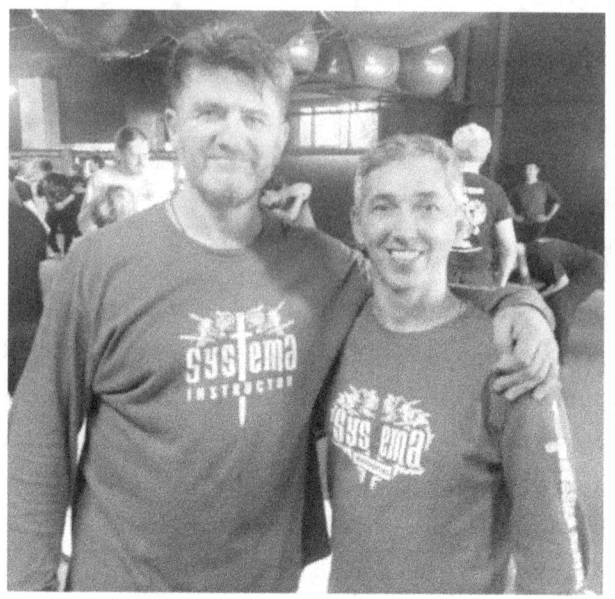

doubted him, I chose to listen to what we was saying. He introduced me to movement, theatre, dance, therapy and many other things that I didn't know it existed.

So I started to study the human body in a broader way and still do. From that I found my other passion: movement. I have three beautiful young boys, they all do sports and martial arts . Now I am a Systema instructor and work as a movement coach and health therapist.

When did you first begin training?

I started to train martial art at age 12, but my father taught me some moves before that, so I wouldn't get beat up so much. I did some boxing, Karate, Kung fu, Krav Maga and Ninjutsu. But basically I was only trying to find a way to survive and beat up others! Then I discovered Aikido and decided to train it but the problem was that the only school was in São Paulo, about 70 km away. So I started to train after work, get the bus for two hours to get to the training area, then two hours to get back. Most of the time I didn't sleep at all.

It was through Aikido that I learned that I didn't need to beat up anyone, that there was more in martial art than just being strong. I wanted to show people what I was learning and decided to open the first school of Aikido in my city, Santos. Shortly after that I started to give classes to police officers, military agents, prison guards and federal agents both in Santos and in São Paulo. So my understanding of martial art and self defence has changed as I got more experience and older.

When did you first see Systema and what were you first impressions?

I first saw Systema in 2002, it was a video of military training, while I was researching for more material that I could bring to the officers students. I was looking for a way to teach simpler stuff for self defence. At first I didn't know what it was, or what it was called! At that time I used to translate a journal of Aikido from English to Portuguese and in 2003 saw an article about Systema and Vladimir Vasiliev, promoting an event called Aiki Expo that Vladimir was participating in. I realised that what I had seen on that video was Systema and started to look were I could train or at least get more info. I sent an e-mail to Vladimir and he said that there wasn't anyone training in South America and that I could buy some VHS tapes and start to train. And so I did, with some of my Aikido black belts in Santos, we created a training group.

I thought it was different, I knew I didn't understand it but it called my attention. So I needed to understand it. The movement was fluid, it didn't really look like a military video. The fact that there wasn't a belt system and that more advanced and newer students could train together also called my attention. I had to learn to do that!

Also, as far as I knew from my previous studies, there were no Christian martial arts and this annoyed me, because I didn't want to change my religion. When I saw Systema and started to study it's connection with orthodoxy Church I was pleased!

How did your club develop and when did you first get to train with Vladimir?

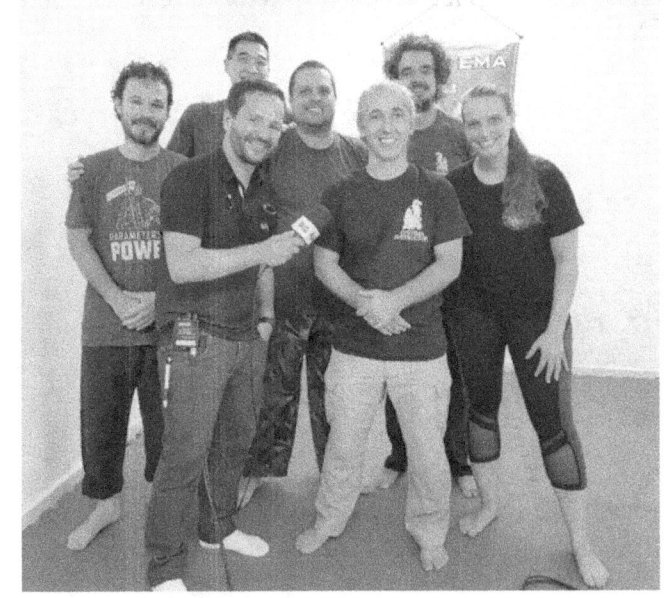

I had a training group with some of my black belt students in Santos and we learned from the videos. A couple of years later a guy from São Paulo, Gustavo Castilhos, reached me, he was also trying to understand Systema. Once a month, or sometimes more he would come to Santos and train with us. We also did some seminars from what we learned from the videos (2005-2006) and then he moved to another country.

One guy from the north of Brazil got my e-mail and asked If I could teach a seminar there, and It was the first time I was on a plane! I thought I understood something about Systema, but I knew I had to go and train with Vasiliev and Ryabko, because there were some things that I was not able to do and I wanted to learn. A student of mine, Fabio, was married to a Danish lady and lived in Denmark, so I decided to make a trip to Europe to stay with them and attend the 2008 *Summit of Masters* in 2008 in Esbjerg . I sold my car and went to my second plane trip! It was an incredible experience. I met people from different parts of the world, visited new countries and could also train!

And from there you were able to expand your club?

Yes, I became a certified instructor and opened the first school of Systema in South America. I was, and still am, determined to show Systema to people, to make my school grow and share all I've learned. I used to teach at Santos and São Paulo. After the trip to Europe I realised that I didn't know so much, so started to bring a certified instructor to teach me and my group as often as I

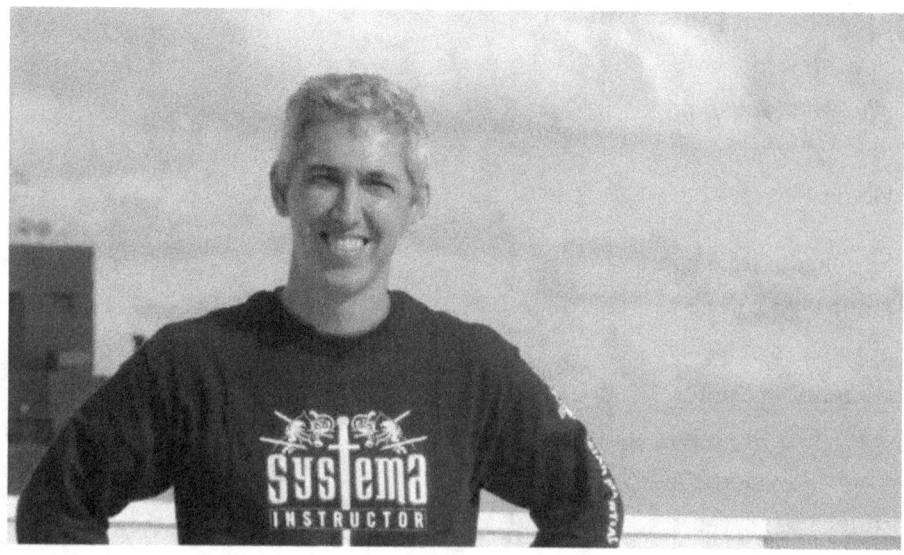

could. He eventually became a good friend for me and this made a huge difference in the quality of our Systema school. I transitioned from a part time to a full time Systema instructor and in 2012 I was able to go for the first time to Toronto and train at HQ. It was awesome! I learned that regular classes are quite different from seminars and did as many classes as I could. In this trip I was also a accompanied by a student that later became an instructor.

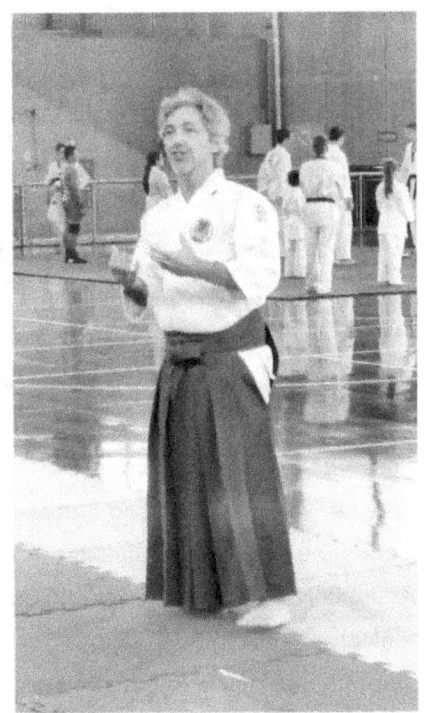

What differences did you find between Systema and your previous training?

In Aikido there are some similarities they talk about relaxation and breathing, there is this idea to control your opponent using his force against him. The talking about principles was similar but the action itself was quite different. Aikido has a focus on the perfect execution of techniques while in Systema the focus is on the application of the concepts and principles.

What, to you, are the defining principles of Systema and how you do put these into your work?

Breathing, relaxation, posture, structure and movement are quite a cliche for being the defining principles of Systema. I found that an interesting principle is human development. If you are training to get strong, you are doing it wrong. If you are training to kill, you are doing it wrong. You should train to develop yourself, to grow, protect. You do that by working through breathing, relaxation, posture/structure and movement. There's no need to do a hundred push ups. You can do only one if you are paying attention to the right place.

You can use physics principles to understand a movement (angle, gravity,

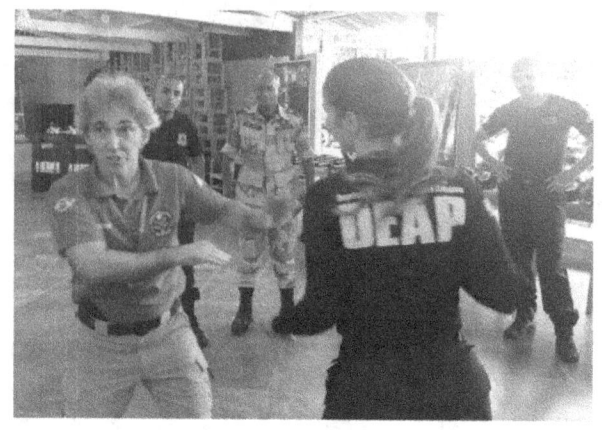

pendulum) but those principles are not only present when you train Systema, they are present in life. If you understand this you will see that you are always training and that you can migrate you training knowledge to other movement areas like in dance.

As Systema is focused more in the principles and concepts, these can and should be used in the full extent of life. I normally say that the only time I stop training is when I am sleeping! You can't unlearn to breath properly, you can't unlearn to move and position your body in your favour. Once, I left the elevator with my backpack, in a rush to go for a class and I slipped in the corridor. The next day I found the concierge looking at the security camera footage because he didn't understand what happened: I recovered my balance so fast and so naturally that he didn't actually believed I slipped when I told him. If your training does not work for life, it is worthless. Why would you do it?

So you find aspects of Systema filter through to all your regular activities?

Systema breathing and the exercises of relaxation can be done in a variety of "real-life" situations, such as when you are stressed in your work. I use Systema in my life and also teach my students to do the same. Most of the people who train will never face a situation where they will have to fight for they life, so when I receive from an older student a feedback that he outpaced his daughter while climbing stairs and had a normal breathing while she was exhausted, this makes me really happy.

When I started to train I wanted to find an easier way to teach. I knew martial arts and self defence, but had only a couple of hours to teach others. Then I saw the philosophy and discovered the health improvement in my own body. I am more interested in the health benefits of Systema nowadays. I'm getting old to kick ass, let the youngsters do that (laughs)!

How do you structure your teaching and how has your teaching style developed?

I work a theme for a week. So if I am doing knife work, I work with it for a week. If I'm doing structure, I work with that for a week. For warm up I work one day with legs, the other day with arms, and so on. I like the basics.

I started to teach Systema because it was easier to teach for the Law Enforcement officers that I worked with. I had only a few hours a week to teach them things that could mean the difference between going back to their homes, to a hospital or to the grave. You don't have to remember, to decorate a sequence of movements, you just understand how your body works and work with it. I already had experienced teaching Aikido and tried my best to not mix them. But I do confess that I took me a while to truly give a Systema class and not an Aikido class with Systema moves.

At first, looking the videos, I tried to copy Vasiliev and Ryabko's movement. Many years later I finally realised I couldn't, because I was not them. I could not move like them because my body was different. I had to find my own way of movement while maintaining the principles. That meant the same for my students; there were trying to copy me or copy a movement. When I started to change the way I teach, my students started to develop much deeper and much faster. I do my best to pass this information for my students, for them to learn with the body they have.

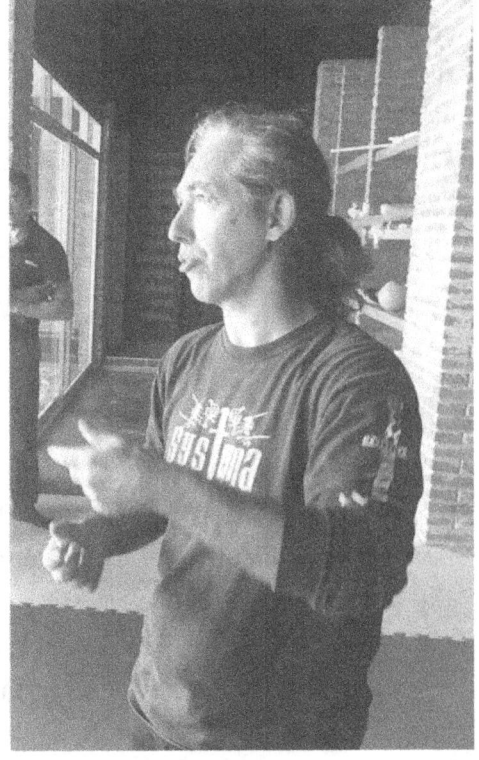

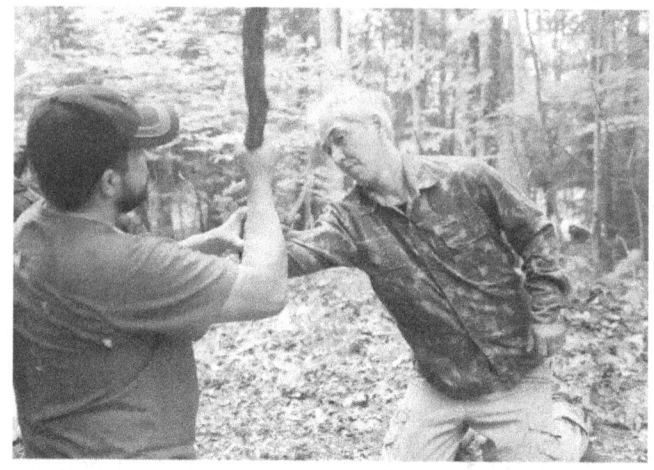
I changed the way I teach over the years. I came to Systema because I found it easier to teach, the philosophy made me open my vision, and I stayed for the health benefits that I gained. So my training also changed from "self-defence" to a more health practice.

Have you also found teaching to be a learning experience in itself?

Yes, because teaching really demands that the principles be clear to yourself. Sometimes, you think you know something and when you have to teach it you realise you didn't know as well as you thought! It's a challenge to guide your students through their own path of self improvement. Don't try to rush it, everyone has their own time to deal with stuff. As Vladimir once said: "Don't take anything from a person without giving something to replace it with".

I try to offer a good environment for my students, a safe place were they can get in touch with their deepest emotions and, maybe, replace them with joy.

How about when you are working with a new group, how do you approach that?

When I go to somewhere new I often ask what they want to learn (sometimes in regular class as well) and see how many students are there. I start with some breathing and movement exercise, which gives me an idea of how well the group can move, how flexible they are, what restrictions and limitations they have, and helps "break the ice." From there I go on to combative techniques. It's a good challenge to use the "warm up" as a part of the technique itself and normally most people don't even realise it. So, if they want to understand more about strikes, I do a lot of push ups, correct the position of the hand, shoulder, how to properly activate the shoulder muscles and the position of the trunk and pelvis.

When the group is new they start to punch in the right way, not only because they are tired, but because their body has then already learned the way to push. I found this way to be way easier than keep asking for a new group to relax, strike while exhaling and so on.

What advice would you give to new Instructors?

For the new instructors, it's important to keep training. Becoming an instructor is not a static position, there's always more to learn. Don't try to do something that you don't feel comfortable with. Go basic when you don't know what to do. The class is not a place for you, as an instructor, to experiment. It is a place for your students to develop their creativity.

What is your view today on Systema, has it changed from when your first saw and experienced it?

I think that Systema is alive and, as something that is alive, it changes, evolves with time. I have been following the change from VHS to DVD to Youtube and even Facebook / instagram. For example, Vladimir's movement has improved over the years, who am I to stay stuck in one place then? Nowadays I understand

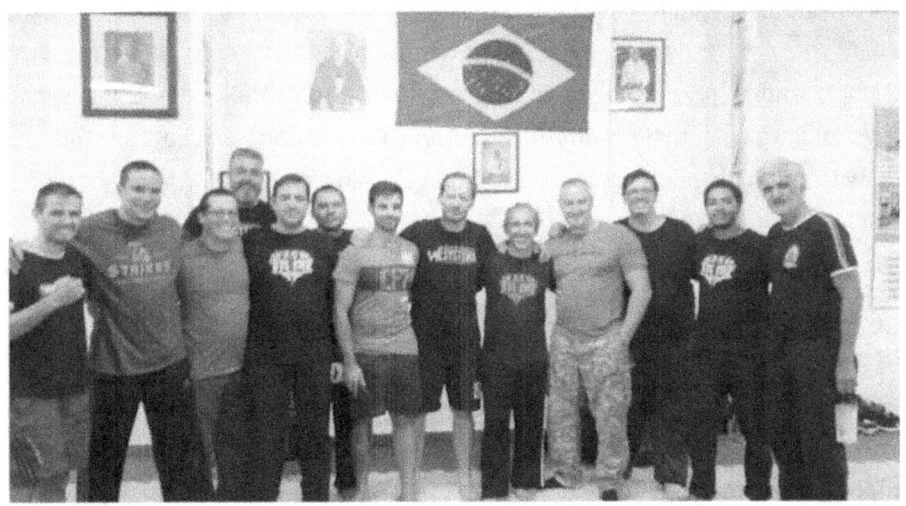

Systema as a tool for self development, where you can see through your own veils, truly feel your emotions and learn to let go of anger and fear, become a better human being. I guess that you only stop to improve yourself when you die and I am not planning to die anytime soon, so I better keep improving!

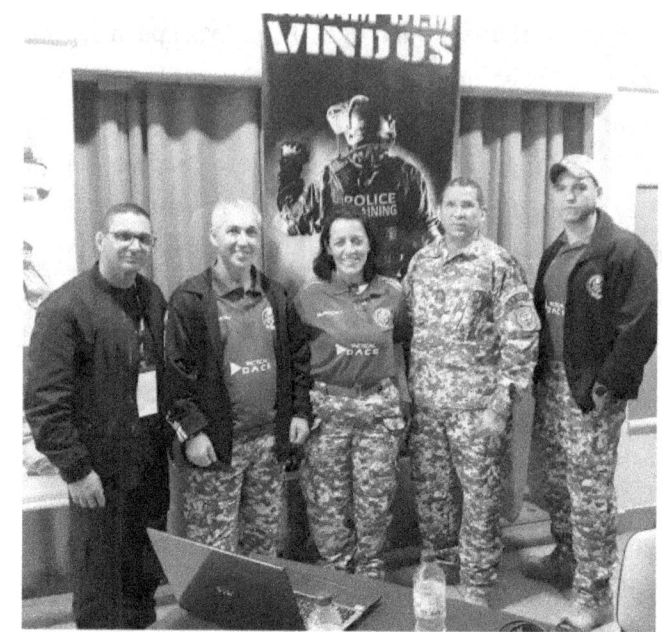

What has Systema brought you?

Systema became my profession. It gave me the opportunity to travel, meet people from all around the world and make friends, do things that I never even dreamed of. I was kindly invited to Peru by Sandro to give seminar there and it was a very nice experience; I can give classes in English and Spanish. I honestly don't know were I would be if I didn't know Systema. My focus on my own training and in my school is to promote health (physically, emotionally and psychologically). It really is amazing to offer the tools and see what the students do with them, developing and growing, to see how they really became free.

Do you have any interesting experiences you would like to share?

One of my best stories is from the first time I met Vladimir and Mikhail in Denmark. Me and my student were from Brazil, the farthest that someone has travelled for that seminar. And when we went out for dinner the people (not only Vladimir and Mikhail but also the students) let us sit in a place close to them, because we had travelled so far. That was something unthinkable for me then, in traditional Eastern martial arts you never sit close to the master because its reserved for the oldest students. That was a huge impact on me and made me realise that there was much more than martial arts in the training, there was a self improvement going on.

In the *Summit of Masters*, Mikhail also showed how to control the heartbeat and synchronize the rhythm with music. He also taught me to breath while praying. It may not sound so special, but it was for me. The ability to control your heart with breathing was something totally new for me. After the seminar I understood that I had a lot to learn!

What do you like to do outside of Systema?

When I am not looking at videos of Systema I am looking at videos of movement and exercises. Apart from the movement community, I like to do outside sports and activities such as tracking. I like to read, eat good food and go to the movies, mostly action ones.

And do you have any final thoughts or advice for the reader?

Never stop learning. Be curious!

SYSTEMA VOICES

CANADA

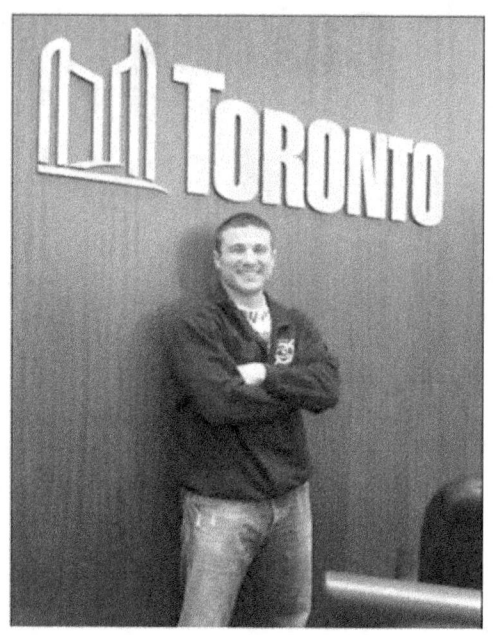

EMMANUEL MANOLAKAKIS

Can we start with your background and where you're from?

My parents emigrated from Greece to Toronto, Canada where I was born and raised. I was a very athletic child and did a lot of sports. I did mostly rugby in high school, as well as American football and baseball. Oddly enough, being a Canadian, I never did play hockey (laughs), mostly due to time restraints.

How did you get into martial arts? What were the first influences and styles?

There were only two types of martial arts available here in Toronto when I first started at age 15. There was traditional Karate and Taekwondo. I choose Karate, which was a form of Shotokan, called Shorin-ryu where I trained for about 2-3 years. Coincidentally I was also wrestling at this time. In my mind I had a difficult time seeing Karate fairing well against wrestling. It was surprising how tough wrestlers were, as well as strong and resilient. I wasn't very confident that my ground training in Karate would help me much in wrestling. I would ask my teachers questions about this and they didn't really know how to answer it nor truly understand my questions at that level.

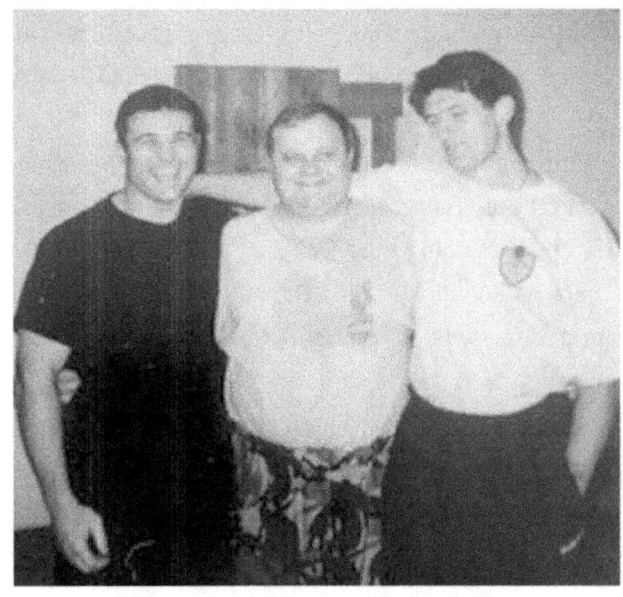

I loved Karate and it's formal discipline.

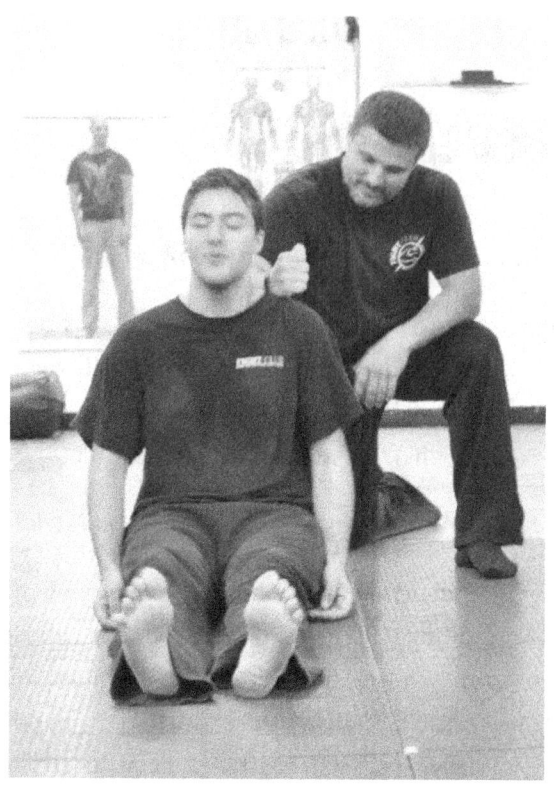

Wrestling, however, was such a stark contrast, it was such a different expression.

Where did you first see Systema and what were your first impressions?

I was training competitively in rugby at York University and had incredible access to Olympic level facilities and trainers. Between my studies, my job, and training, I didn't have much time for martial arts. Once I graduated, I was drawn back to the martial arts. There was a brief time that I boxed and really enjoyed the intensity of the training, but had no desire to box professionally. I also had no desire to pursue a martial art that had a belt system, which I found to be frustrating.

A friend of mine from University called me up one day, saying he had heard about this Russian guy in Richmond Hill, that was opening up a martial arts school. He advertised no belts, no uniforms, and no katas. At that time, no one was doing this. So I went to go check out this Russian martial art and there was Vlad. He didn't speak much English but was very welcoming and interacting with everybody. You could work with the instructor and ask him questions. This was very different from the other martial arts. You couldn't get close to the top teachers, that was unheard of. Vlad showed us stuff that I had never seen before. He would dismantle the body in such a natural way. I left after my first class saying, "I want to do more of this. This is awesome."

What sort of things were you training in those early classes?

The first class was focused on hand-to-hand combat. My second class, he was showing a multiple attacker scenario. I had played a lot of rugby in high school and at university, so I knew what happened when a lot of guys got together and there was some kind of disagreement. I had an idea of multiple attack fighting. When Vlad was talking about this scenario I was listening and thought to myself, "This guy knows exactly what he's talking about and from first hand experience." I didn't know too many people that had that experience. I left that class just amazed and invigorated. I never thought you could teach or methodically understand a mass fight, I always had thought it was just chaotic. Vlad actually showed how you could survive in that situation, as well as understand it. I drove home after class and thought either Vlad is crazy or what he's teaching me is incredibly masterful and deep. There is a lot that we don't understand about Systema. We just keep training and going deeper and deeper into its applications.

So it was very different from the other arts around, at the time?

Yes, because in Toronto back then, the environment was saturated with katas and formalities that the traditional martial arts promote. And then you have a guy like Vlad that comes in that says just punch, kick, and grab me and we will figure this out. You had this perfect storm of people tired of the traditional stuff and wanting something new. And then the excitement of Vlad coming in and showing it. We were like kids eating fruit...we didn't have the understanding that comes from a tree or its roots. We were just enjoying the fruit.

So what was it that prompted you to begin teaching and how did you find that at first?

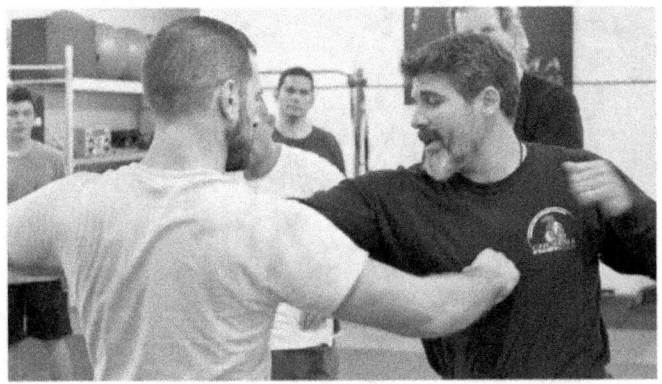

Well, It kind of happened slowly as I trained over

the years. I was very dependable and consistent in my training. When a teacher sees a consistency in you, he's able to build and construct something because he knows you're around to break it down and build it back up. I started leading the class in the warm up. It was an honour to lead the warm ups and get the guys ready for Vlad. It just kept going deeper and deeper. One day Vlad said, "If you really want to understand Systema, it is good to teach it." The ultimate form of knowing is teaching. I saw value in this and would teach classes when there was an opportunity. I never had any ambitions to start my own school and was very content training and teaching at Vlad's. When I got married, my wife and I decided to move to East York which made for quite a commute to the school, especially with starting up a family. Vlad advised me to start my own school and get up to train with him when I could. So I found a little space, started Fight Club, and expected it only to be a part-time thing. It was so small, less then 1000 square feet in a basement. I had about 5-6 students and we trained 2 times a week. The school just kept growing and I had to move to a bigger facility. Within three or four years I outgrew that. I ended up having two full-time jobs at that time. It kept growing until I quit my other job and committed myself to teaching Systema at Fight Club full time 10 years ago.

I understand you have experience in coaching different disciplines, could you tell us something about that? And also, what crossover you've found from teaching Systema and coaching?

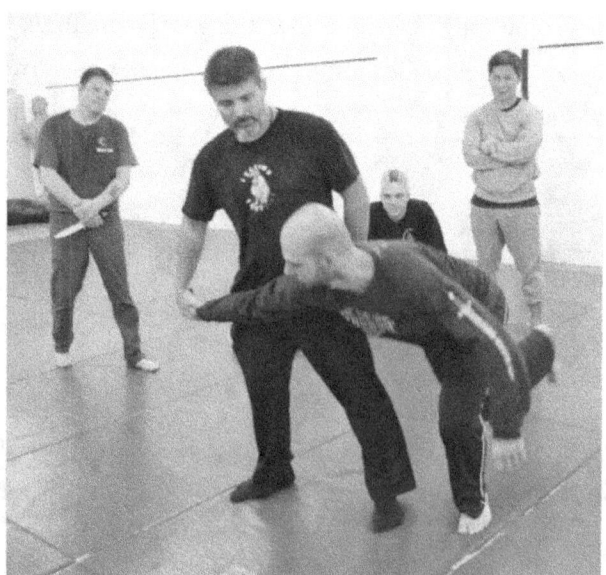

Coaching, teaching, and motivating are all one in the same. First you understand the sport and the rules. Then you motivate people to get to that point. Coaches would

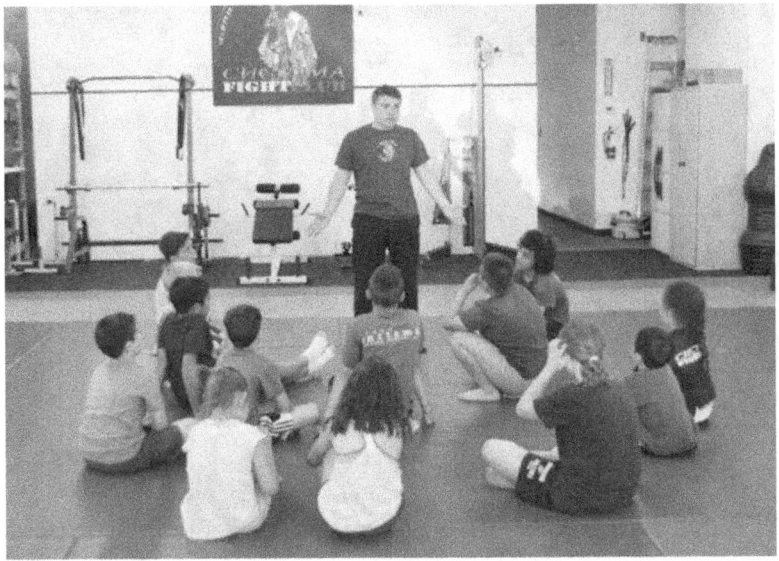

come to the Fight Club and ask me to work with their team with team building, communication, focus, and toughness. So with the toughness, for example, I'm working with their ability not to give up despite the circumstances they are faced with within their specific sport. All those exercises in Systema where we are doing push ups on each other and moving with people lying on top of you, they all help with that. And, of course, even just the breathing alone is immense. I've been asked specifically to help with breathing and enable the athletes to make calm and collected decisions. Some of the exercises we do in groups, if you take the fighting out of it, I find that they help significantly with team building and trust.

I coach my daughter's soccer team from the Systema aspect. One drill I use is to have a person come at you with a stick and you simply have to move out of the way. This teaches the soccer players how to move. So you study how to move your body away from danger. In the game you're moving your body away from the opponent into an open space to get to the ball. Another drill I use is where you are moving on the ground with someone on top of you and getting comfortable with contact. There is contact in all sports. Any player can use these concepts to handle contact, not be fearful of it, and be moving effectively with it. Systema is useful no matter what the sport because it includes the physical, mental, moving, breathing, and how they all relate to performance.

As you continue in Systema, do you appreciate more the depth of training?

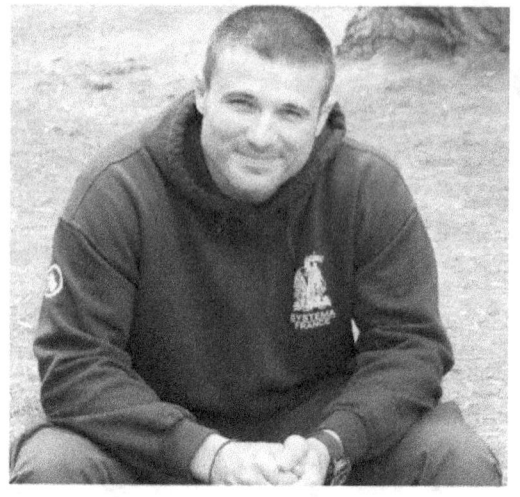

One hundred percent! Personally I don't believe we have even seen half of Systema. I find that the deep aspects of Systema are in everything and believe there's just so much more to it than what you see on the surface, especially at the professional level of any sport. At the amateur level, people can get away with just talent. As you get to the upper levels of most sports, you cannot get by with just talent. You have to get more polished. This is where the art of Systema comes in.

When you go somewhere new and teach a new group of people, how do you organize the training?

A teacher can only truly teach to the average of the room. You have to look at the common denominator and teach to that. A teacher has to take the group through a general overview of everything. Get them moving, breathing, doing the basic exercises, and working together. You have to be attentive. Just observe the skill, understanding, behaviour, fear, and ego within the group. Make sure they have a good foundation and that what you are building is solid. If I were to use a pyramid as an example, the wider the base of the pyramid the higher the peak can be.

Do you have any advice to instructors on how to structure their sessions?

For new instructors, there's a lot of information out there. Books, videos, YouTube, and newsletters, that are easily at your disposal. Make sure you're accessing it. Keep yourself up to date. Study teaching, leadership, and motivation. Learning Systema is one thing. Teaching Systema is another thing.

Take the time to read about just teaching. Then learn how to teach Systema on whatever site is relative to you. Learn from the videos. This is an ongoing thing that needs to be done weekly. Then there's your own training, we all have something to work on. You have to be open to change and grow. If students see you learning and growing, they will follow your example. When you go to seminars, ask other instructors questions, ask them about teaching. Some seminars have days specifically for instructors. Network and get to know other instructors. I think there's now enough information out there to get anyone started.

How do you feel Systema has developed over the years?

In the early years of Systema, it was not as well defined. By that I mean there was little breath work, not a lot of push ups or squat drills. We just came to class and studied self defence. Vladimir had so much energy and was very excited to show this art to whomever wanted to learn. It has changed over the years. If you really want to understand something in a masterful way, you have to go deeper. Re-understand what you know and grow. As the years went on, more details were discovered. It has been distilled year after year, with a finer and smoother product. The depth of Systema has just been fabulous to witness in my many years of training. As the years went on, like with anything, the newness wore off and we start training deeper. You have to go back to the

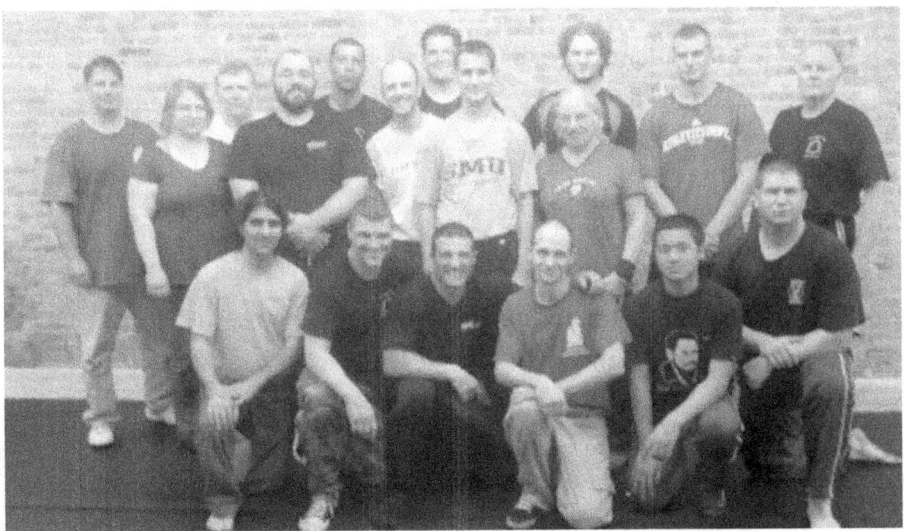

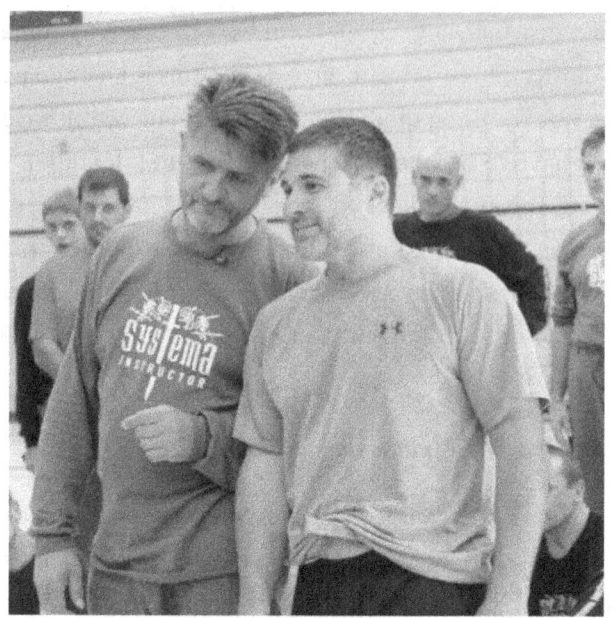

beginning and re-invent yourself. Any athlete develops a level of proficiency. Let's say I'm a hockey player and I develop my skills as a junior. I have a skill and a way of practicing that when I'm 10 years old worked for me. When I got older, maybe what I did then doesn't work anymore. I have to re-invent my hockey and my skills to go deeper. My shots need to be harder and my skating needs to be faster. It's not practicing harder, its getting smoother. Systema is the same way. Over the years you will see how different things were introduced and how the results went deeper. This is important. Systema is a living process. Its amazing how it's developing and it's nowhere near finished. There's so much deeper we can go.

Do you have any good stories to share about Mikhail and Vladimir?

Within the first month of meeting Vlad back in 1994, we were doing some knife work. At one point, Vladimir hit the knife out of his opponent's hand and the knife fell on the ground between the two of them. They both looked at each other like who's going to go for the knife. Vlad stepped on it with his bare foot. He grabbed it between his toes, then lifted his leg and put the knife to the student's neck. Between the creativity, the level of skill, and dexterity that this took...I was just amazed. The ability to even see the option of picking up the weapon in such a manner showed me the level of mastery that Vlad had.

With Mikhail, it was different. He came to Toronto for a seminar and there was one student that came from Australia, named David Quail. At one point in the seminar, Mikhail wanted to work with him since he had come all that way.

As David got close, Mikhail looked up at him and then put his hand up in a stopping position. At that point, David stopped. Mikhail walked closer to David, gave him a big hug, and whispered something to him. David started crying. It was a really uncomfortable moment for all of us to watch this. We didn't even know what Mikhail said. I remember looking over at Vlad and he raised his hands up and didn't know what to make of it either. David explained to everyone what had happened.

David had served in the military special forces. During the demo, Mikhail told him, "You haven't come home yet." David realized that people had told him this before. Due to his respect for Mikhail, however, this meant a lot to him and he knew it must be true. This was profound. To me, I saw a happy-go-lucky Australian guy, not aggressive or angry at all. Mikhail could see through all of that. It's mind-blowing to speak to the level of skill Mikhail works at and how deep he goes with a person. Both Mikhail and Vlad show incredible skills in different ways that just further show the depth of what Systema can do.

You recently wrote something about letting the other person work physically while you worked to suppress your ego. This is a difficult area for most of us. What are your thoughts?

You will get partners that will teach you a lot about yourself in many ways. I trained at Vlad's about a month ago and had an inexperienced partner that was in the mindset of using tension to "win." He was just hell bent on physically dominating me. Physically, I gave him just enough tension, but not as much as what he was giving me. Psychologically, I

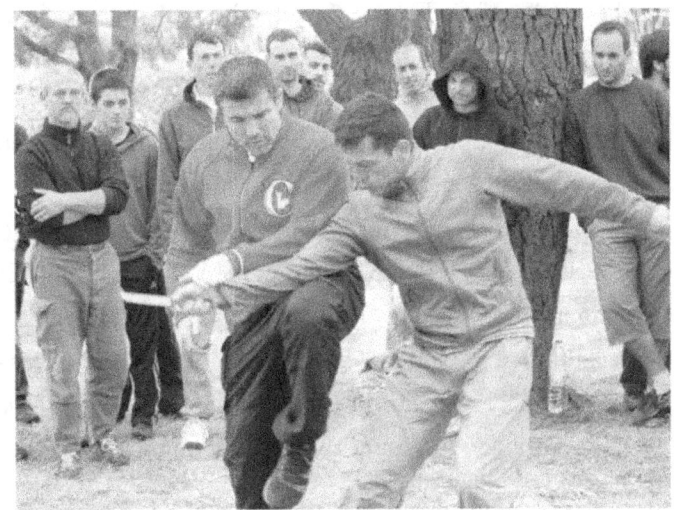

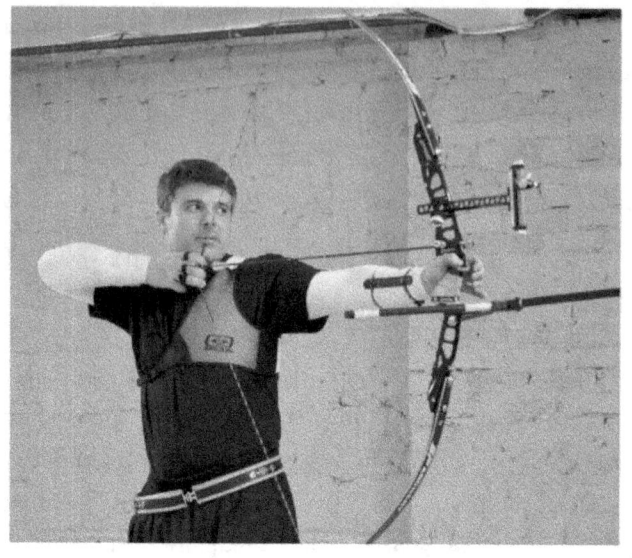

don't upset myself and I try not to further upset my partner. This is an interesting place. Thirdly, I want this whole experience to have a positive effect on the both of us. I want the person who is really tense, to become more relaxed.

So I'm working on three levels and trying my hardest to do so. As the exercise went on, my partner was just getting more tired and agitated. I started to see my ego pop up. I could turn this and quickly choke this person or grab an arm bar. I realized that if I just trained to dominate someone that upset me, then I go right back to the beginning and start all over again. It's similar to someone that is trying to diet and avoid sugar. There's a point where you just need to not eat those things so you don't regress. People start to eat good for a week or two, then all of a sudden they have one day where they eat cake. Then they go right back to their old habits. In Systema, we have a lot of old habits. Systema is much more than a martial art, its about who I am. Was my partner able to accomplish anything? Not really... we were at a stale-mate to be perfectly honest.

In training, people will frustrate and upset you. This is the real work. There's power in relaxation. There's power in calmness. This is more then just an idea, you have to work with this concept against tense and strong people.

In class I watch a really good person meet a really bad person. Watch the two meet, who will win here? Will the good person make the bad person good? Or will the bad person make the good person bad? You see this in business, in a street fight...you see this happen all the time. Who will influence who? If you want to be a good person, then study being a really good person and study how to make a bad person good.

I see that you also enjoy archery and fishing. Are these hobbies you have been involved in for awhile?

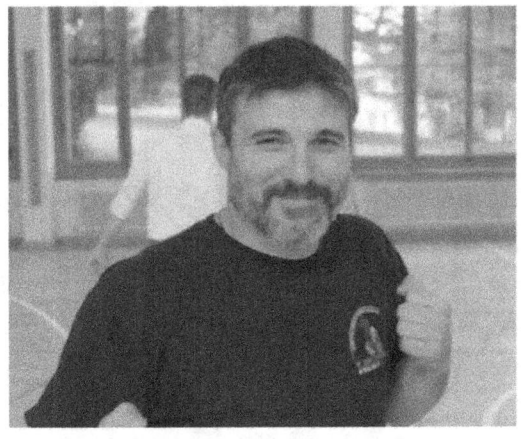

I've been fishing since I was a young boy and enjoy it quite a bit. It's very relaxing to be on the water and around good friends. This is definitely a great hobby for me. Archery, on the other hand, is so much more. I went to a range about seven years ago and picked up a bow. I fell in love right away and have been training archery ever since. Archery is a very internal art and has so much crossover with Systema. So much of it is relaxation, comfort, and not anticipating. It takes a high degree of skill. You see people training for 20-30 years and still learning. I think archery is something I'm going to do for the rest of my life, much like Systema. I liked it so much that I offer it at Fight Club and it has a huge following.

What does Systema mean to you now? And what do you think the future holds for yourself?

Konstantin once said, "Systema will not live your life for you. You have to live your life." I often think about Systema as a good walking stick. When you stumble or get tired, the stick is there for you to give you support and safety. I realize the depths of Systema and the work I have on myself is a lifelong journey. I use Systema like a good stick in the many aspects of my life. If anyone has gone on a long hike, you realize how simple and important this thing is. I'm constantly training and re-understanding myself everyday. This is never-ending.

Systema has such unbelievable growth. It's nowhere near its full potential. There is a tremendous aspect in teaching this martial art and a responsibility to teach it properly in its entirety. I try to express this to all my students so that they too can understand it. My future is teaching Systema, but also helping teachers become great teachers. My passion is to share my knowledge of

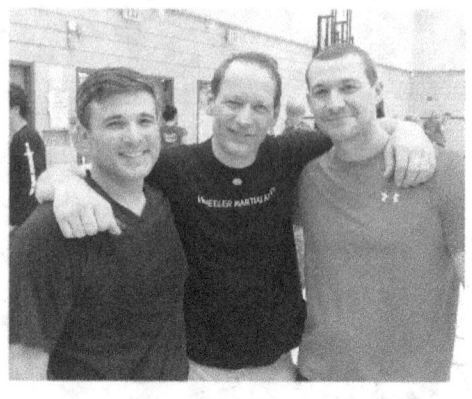

teaching as well as it's implications with Systema. When I look back to 25 years ago, there was just one school. Now look at how many schools and instructors there are. There are billions of people on this planet. Of these people, how many could benefit from Systema? On a smaller scale, look at the city you live in. How many people could you share the gift of Systema with? The biggest challenge that Systema has is getting the people to come train. Show them what Systema can do for them and I guarantee they will stay. Everybody should know about it. We all say the same thing about Systema, "I wish I had known about it sooner." Get the people through the doors and they will see for themselves.

Lastly is there anything you would like to add for our readers? Any advice or thoughts?

There are three things I want people to understand. First, when you're just training the martial art of Systema, you are only training 15-20%. There is also Systema of your family. The problems that exist in you as a martial artist, will also manifest themselves within your family. Then there's Systema of your work, your job, and your career. Whatever plagues you on the mats, will eventually come up at work as well.

There's Systema of your hobbies and of your general health. You can look at all the different aspects and divide it as you like. If my profession is a doctor and telling people bad news brings me great tension, causes me stress or sadness, then I need to use Systema to help me deal with that so I can be a better doctor. I have to understand and deal with these problems. Every job has it's arm bars, every family life has it's headlocks. Every aspect of our lives has interpretations in the martial arts. So if you can't breath when you're doing martial arts, you're going to be holding your breath at home when dealing with a stressful situation. Start training Systema while you're at home and look at how you interact with your family. Try to get rid of tension, build understanding, communicate and work together. Now you are training Systema at home. The more time I can I can commit to doing something, the quicker and deeper I am going to understand it. If you want to fully understand Systema and get the most out of it, look at your home life, your family, your work, your hobbies, and apply your training to them.

Secondly, when I'm teaching people, I try to really build them, their skills and their understanding. I believe that Mikhail and Vlad only teach to the average of our understanding. If one day when we are at a seminar and everyone there is focused, has done their homework, practiced diligently, worked on their breathing and movement, then they, in turn, are going to start giving us more. And we are going to go even deeper into Systema together. If we just keep attending seminars and beating the hell out of each other, I truly think we won't see as much as we think because we will not be ready for it. We have to show our teachers that we are ready. When we come to training, we must do our best to prepare ourselves. Work hard on the mental, physical, and spiritual aspects of yourself. Make sure they are all as good as you can get them. And that will be good enough.

Thirdly, in many cases the most fruitful learning is when people take the time to truly appreciate each other. When you train, get to know each other and work on each other. You can beat on a person and do so much more when he knows you understand him. Whenever Vlad or Mikhail has worked with me, there's an incredible amount of appreciation we have for each other. I don't ever feel like they are trying to hurt me or trying to prove something, they are only trying to teach me.

I know that this is hard when you get difficult training partners, but you've got to take the time to understand each other's perspective, goals, and hopes. This is such a humane martial art and I wish people would practice this more. That doesn't mean training soft. I hit hard when I work with people, but its humane. It's from the inside out. If you appreciate each other, I think you will find a deeper and better form of learning.

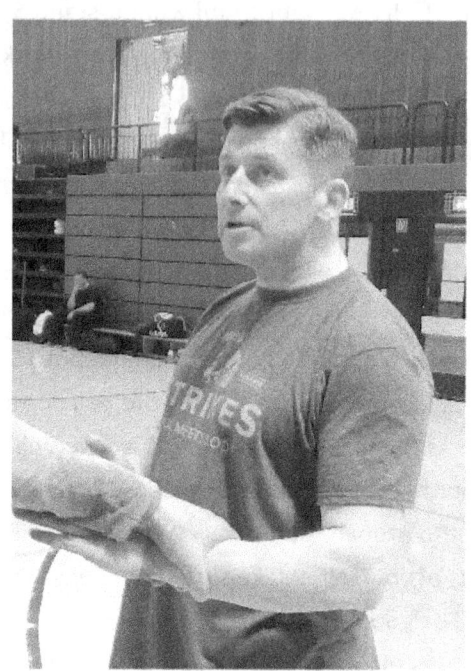

JASON PRIEST

Can we start with something about your background?

I grew up on the East coast of Canada on an Air Force base, my dad was in the services. The local town was small, just around ten thousand people. For High School you had to be bussed, it was about half an hour to the local High School. Not a lot went on there, there weren't a lot of martial art schools like you'd find in a big city. There was one local Taekwondo school, that was it. Martial arts was something I'd had an interest in since I was young, but I think at the time I couldn't have afforded the lessons.

So when did you first start training in martial arts?

Well later on, to put myself through University I moved to South Korea to teach English. I was there for three years, off and on, to make some money. It was a big move, at the time South Korea wasn't like it is today. There were not so many foreign visitors, not too many people spoke English but I had a friend who had moved there before me. So he helped me get set up, introduced me around. It was a bit of a culture shock, there were some ups and downs but it's the good parts you remember (laughs).

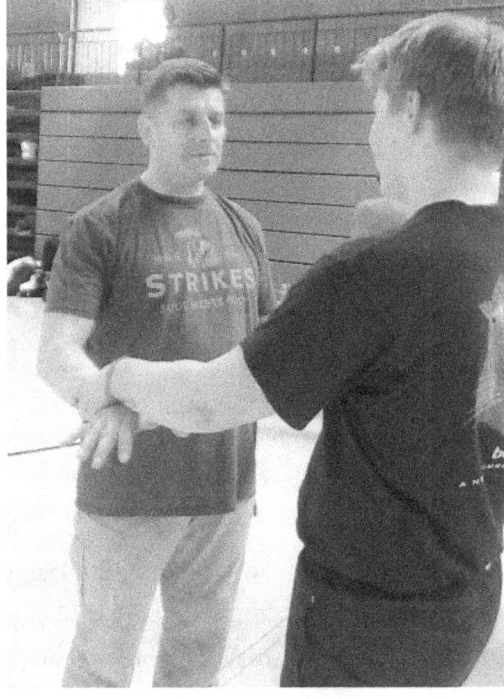

I started training in Taekwondo there, I did that for quite some time. These days TKD is more sports based. There are

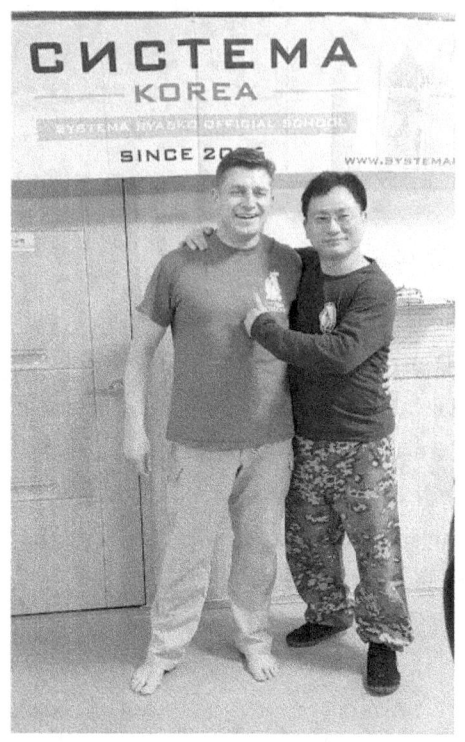

still some schools around in Korea that teach the old, hardcore style but for the most part it's three minute rounds, pads, points, WTF Olympic style. It was good exercise, you know you fancy yourself as being a martial artist after you've been in it for a while. But even back then, before I was introduced to Systema, I used to stop and think once in a while what my capabilities might be. I mean I'm not the sort of person who gets into fights and trouble, I try and fly under the radar as much as I can, but I didn't feel that any of the work I'd done was of any real value for self defence. It's a little like Mikhail was saying this morning, for some styles everything has to be just right. Whether it's a second or two to prepare yourself, the circumstances, your distancing and so on.

So you began to question the training?

Yes because, you know, I had some grand ideas about what it meant to be a martial artist. I think inside everybody there's a little bit of a desire to be the hero, to protect themselves, their family and friends. Since I started Systema I think I lost some of that feeling (laughs). To be a hero, I mean.

What was your first exposure to Systema and what were your first impressions?

Growing up on a base as I did and with the Cold War still on, we were told that the Russian nukes were targeted on us, because we had the planes that track submarines stationed nearby. So you kind of grew up with this idea that the Russians were scary, capable of doing anything. But I'd never heard of any

Russian martial arts until I was in the grocery store one day and was flipping through a copy of Black Belt magazine. There was an ad in there for Vladimir's DVDs, in particular it was the ones for knife and gun defence. In TKD we had never done any work like that, so I thought Spetsnaz, well these guys seem pretty tough and know what they're doing, maybe I'll check this out. I went on the website and ordered the DVDs but it hadn't clicked to me that these guys were in Toronto.

A couple of weeks later this box turned up with a Toronto return address on it but no name, it didn't say Russian Martial Art or anything. I was wondering what it was, what had I ordered from Toronto? Of course it was the DVDs, plus some flyers for the school. As soon as I realised they were so close, I thought I have to go up and see these guys.

Were you still training in TKD at the time?

Yes and the school I was at had started bringing in a BJJ guy once a week, just so you could get a little bit of cross-training in ground work. There was a flyer in with my DVDs about a ground work seminar Vladimir was teaching in Montreal so I thought I'd go to that, it would be a good comparison. But first I thought it would be good to take a couple of classes at Toronto, to get a feel for it. So I visited and the first class was just amazing. I had a couple of classes and a couple of private sessions then did the workshop. I don't think I've ever been hit so much in my life as I was at that seminar (laughs). At one point you stop and think *What am I doing here*, you know? But then you think, well okay, this isn't so bad, I'm learning about

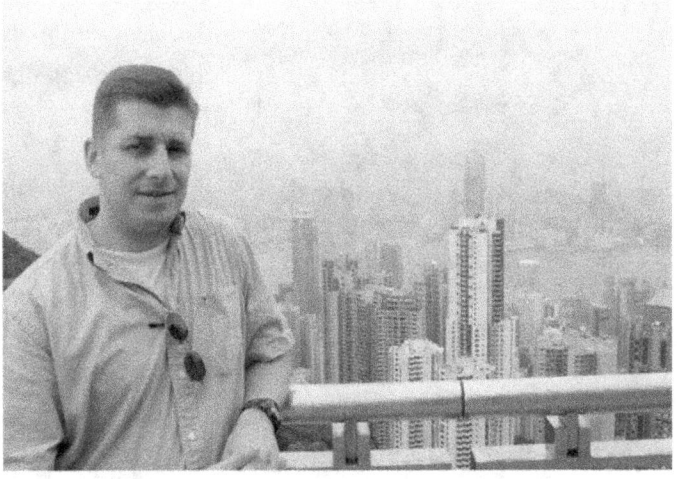

myself, so you stay. I've been loving it ever since, I've been training regularly now for about twelve years.

Did you feel, like many of us, that whatever you had trained in before had not really prepared you for that first Toronto session?

Yes, in many ways your previous experience kind of sets you up to get knocked down. You have some ideas in your head about what you are capable of and then you learn very quickly there's a whole lot you are not prepared for, or capable of! But I think if you go in with the attitude to learn, that's not a deterrent, it's an eye opener. You see that there is a much bigger world out there, interesting things to learn, new ways to grow and develop and that's what I thought was really fantastic.

All my years in TKD, you learn under people who have been doing it a long time, 7th degree back belts and the like. But by the time they get to that point they are more about running their schools. You can see as the years go by and

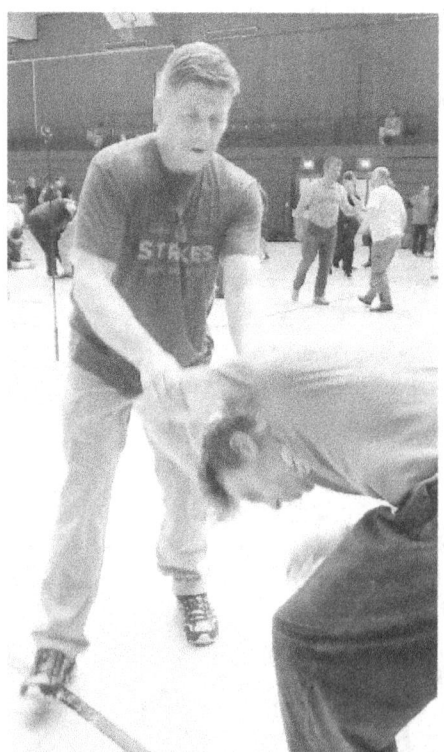

you progress that you get much closer to their skill level, right? But with Vladimir the thing that impressed me most, and what you notice after several years training with him, is that he constantly improves. You never really catch up with him, if anything he is accelerating, the gap might be even bigger now (laughs).

And you don't notice your own progression so much?

Right, it's only when you work with new people that you start seeing what you can do. But you can also see how much further you have to go. It's a very humbling martial art but not in a negative way. A lot of people associate humbling with being embarrassed, or defeated somehow in public but in Systema it's not that kind of humbling, it's more in the sense of you see how much there is still left to learn. That's a pretty cool thing, because it doesn't matter if people are in 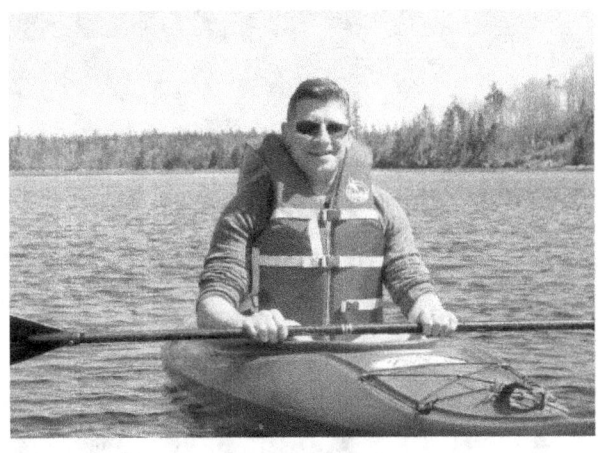 martial arts or studying in a school, or even their job, it shows that there may be new levels to work to, new heights to attain.

Do you think that Systema itself is still developing, it isn't set in stone?

Yes and I think it's because what Systema really boils down to is understanding yourself as a person, how you fit into this world and into humanity in general. Those things are ever-changing so you start to see the limitless potential of what it is to be a human being. Very few of us ever achieve our full potential, maybe very few ever will, but how many ever really try? They get to a certain level and fall into routines, begin to coast. This is something that you feel you can always use to improve yourself, somehow.

In that sense Systema is about developing our full potential?

Well a big thing you hear Mikhail and Vladimir talk about is opening ourselves up. Not just physically but emotionally, mentally and spiritually. To accept what is around you without fighting it, without closing ourselves off, without judgement, really. So you adapt, you move, you flow with what goes on and I think once people get in that groove, they are able to make better use of their talents. They don't let things shut them down. You often run into people who get discouraged, maybe they've had a series of hardships in their life, more and more they close themselves off. Other people open themselves up. So yes, the more you open up, you'll get knocked around a bit. Even the exercises we

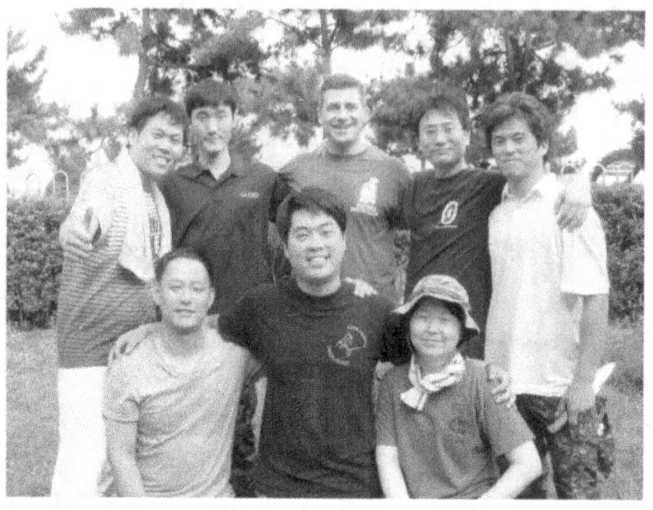
did this morning showed us that as you open up, the knocks come but you use those knocks to energise yourself, right? If you take the negativity and lock it into yourself it becomes damaging. If you open yourself, you allow that energy to move. If you have the right attitude, you can put it back out in a more constructive fashion.

That way you can influence the people around you?

Yes, you can see that by the influence Vladimir has had on the people who come to train. After a while their lives change, and they appear completely different. Some of them come in quite shy, now they are talking to everyone, people become more positive.

Do you think that has something to do with the way Systema is structured too? It's about sharing experience.

Very much so. As knowledgeable and skilled as Vladimir and Mikhail are, they recognise you can learn from anybody. Many times Vladimir said to me that when new, inexperienced people come in, they are the best to learn from. They have no pre-conceived ideas, so you get to see the true reactions they have to certain things you do, you begin to understand how someone who is not trained can be unpredictable and fast. So you can learn how unprepared you are for things like that. There's always a lot to learn from everyone, which is why it's good to work with as many different training partners as you can. It's great to come to an event like this with people from all over the world. I mean, it's wonderful to be in Toronto and be with Vlad all the time but there's always value in training with other people.

A good thing is we have people visiting Toronto all the time from all over, almost every class you meet someone new and get to train with someone from a different background, different levels, and different experiences. But coming out the international seminars you also get to meet the people who aren't always able to come to Toronto. So most of the people here today I've never met before, that's a lot of good opportunities to work with others. You pick up gems, little bits and pieces from all the people you work with.

When did you first start teaching and what have you learned from it?

I do have some teaching experience in my background, I taught finance courses at the University of Toronto for ten years. Not a full credit programme but night school. Prior to that, I did a lot of consulting work in pensions, a few years of presentations and the like, so it's quite natural for me to get up in front of people and talk and show things. The way I first got into it with Systema, is that Frank Arias was going down to South America to do some seminars for the military and police down there. I'd only been training for a few years at the time but thought it would be a pretty cool trip to go on and, as Frank was leading it, there wouldn't be too much responsibility or pressure on my part. That's how

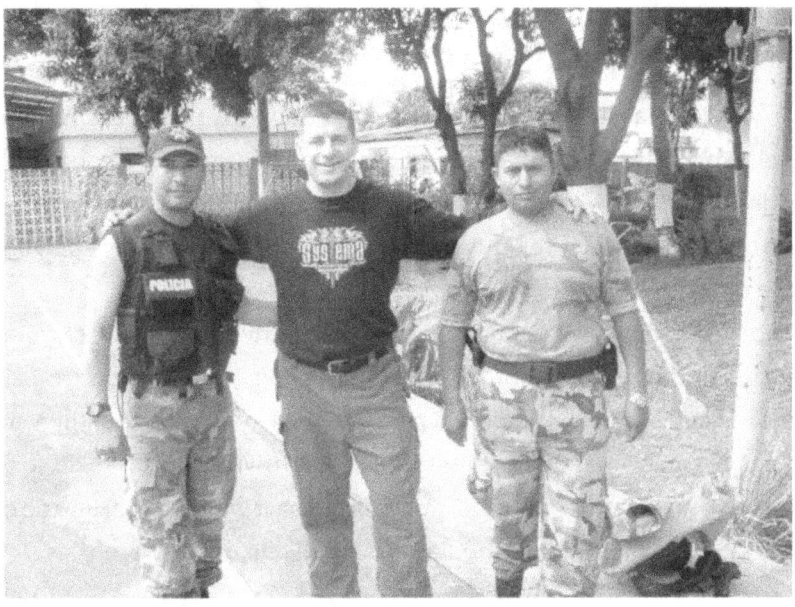

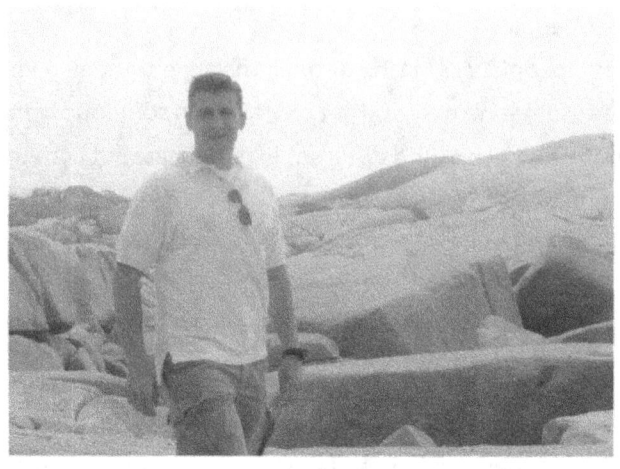

I became an Instructor in Training, that's how it started.

Then I moved on to instructing some of the breathing classes in Toronto when they started, filling in for the kids classes and working my way up. It's a lot of fun. I've learnt a lot through teaching classes, especially when, once you've told everyone what to do for the drill, you get to watch everybody. You have to try and watch the whole group at once, make sure they aren't hurting each other, seeing how you can help. A lot of times, when you do the exercise yourself, you just focus on yourself. When you lead the group, you watch other people and start to recognise tension in them. Before you approach them to correct them, you think a little bit about have you experienced that tension yourself, how did you deal with it? Then you can share that, so I've found my learning has accelerated since I started teaching.

Do you find that awareness continues outside of class?

I try to maintain that, yes, you notice how people walk, for example. At the beginning of class I like to have people walk and breathe. It's good to watch how people walk, where they hold tension, who might have an injury somewhere. If you take the time and have patience you can start applying that outside of class as well.

The best example I can give is when you're driving and you see someone coming up in the rear view mirror. They're not going very fast but you kind of get the feeling that they're going to pass you, pull in front of you, then change lanes again, and it happens. With something like driving, which we do so much, we tend to be taking information in and processing it without thinking too much. Somehow, our minds and our bodies are picking up on all these cues. A lot of time when we train, we think too much and maybe block some of that out. So we need to open ourselves a little more and work on the feeling.

When teaching, how do you maintain a balance between explanation and experience?

I have to be careful that I try not to talk too much, because of my previous background (laughs). There's a lot of value in the different teaching styles in Systema. Vladimir gives direction, then shows by doing something. Everything you need to know, you can see by watching. But people have different learning styles, not everyone has the patience or understanding to gather that. To a large degree you have to let people figure things out for themselves, to feel it. That's the big difference, in other arts I studied everything was laid out this way, or that way, if you wanted to get fancy you put together some combinations. There are certain people who can work through that and figure out their own methods, I guess, they don't just do what someone said. But for the most part, people follow.

The other thing is I have to be mindful that I may be wrong about certain things, so I don't want to give people information that's not correct. Or even if it's generally correct, something that might not be helpful for them directly. So at most I try and explain, when we are doing an exercise, why we are doing it and the things you should be looking out for, rather than, here's a technique, you have to do it this way. Telling people to slow down, watch out for tension here, what the goal is, I've found people have been receptive to that.

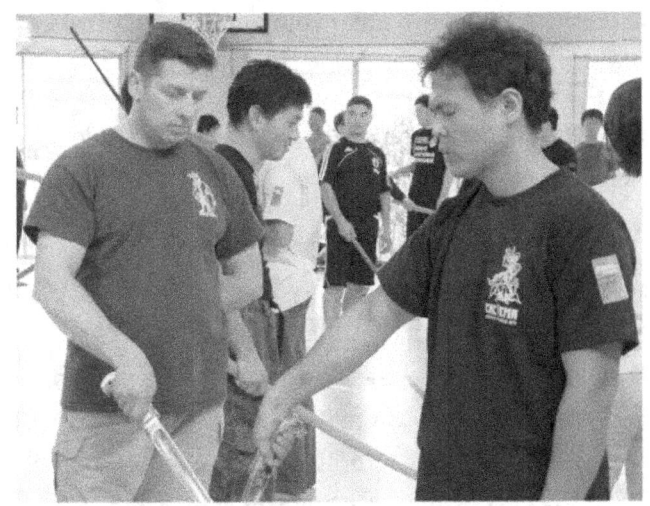

Do you also sometimes find that students come up

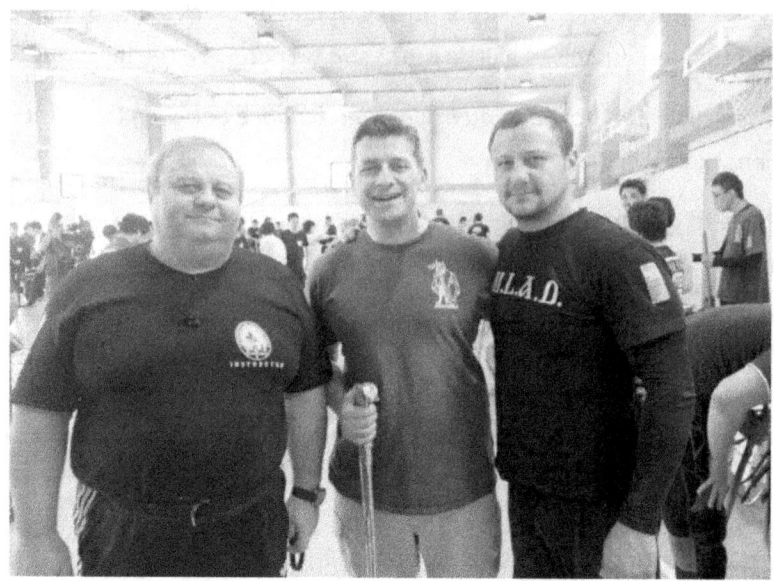

with other angles to drills that you hadn't thought of?

I think we have to remember as individuals, even people with great imaginations, that we can't think of all possibilities, of all concepts. I remember a long time ago, Vlad was running an improvised weapons seminar. He told us how in his military days they'd have a unit of guys sitting round with an umbrella or something. They would pass it around and each one would have to share their ideas about how it could be used. So you might see two things, another person would see two other completely different things. That's the strength of the group approach.

Do you find that people are coming into training with different ideas and expectations these days?

There has been a big change. When I first trained at Toronto you'd have some really tough looking guys coming in, because they'd heard it was Spetsnaz, big guys, muscled up. But they'd have trouble getting through the slow push ups and the like, so it was rare you'd see them for a second class. It tended to be that way, people wanted to see some kind of brutal, fancy martial arts but now it's more people interested in it for their general well being. There's still an interest in the martial art side, of course, but they see the other possibilities as well. The breathing classes have opened the door for that. Some are worried about coming to a martial art class but after trying the breathing class and enjoying it, they see the same teachers are running the other sessions, so they transition over to the martial arts class too.

Do you think that in one sense, Systema is an antidote to our modern reliance on technology?

I think so. In terms of technology cutting us off from other people, it also tends to cut us off from ourselves too, right? The more you stare at a screen, the less you think. I like Systema because it is more raw, it's just people. You don't need special equipment or a special location, even. There's a lot of contact with other people required, it causes you to look both inward and outward at the same time, to be more observant.

What have been the major benefits for you, personally?

It's calmed me down a lot. Any kind of issues, tension from work, relationships, or society in general... even if you just read the news, it can make you tense! So you start to realise how certain things don't matter so much or that you can still have a good life for yourself regardless of what's coming at

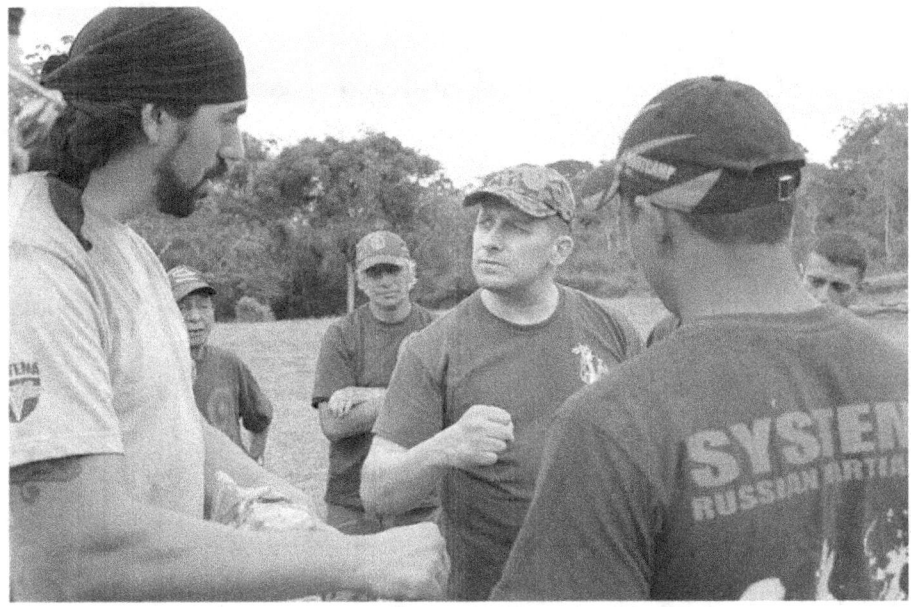

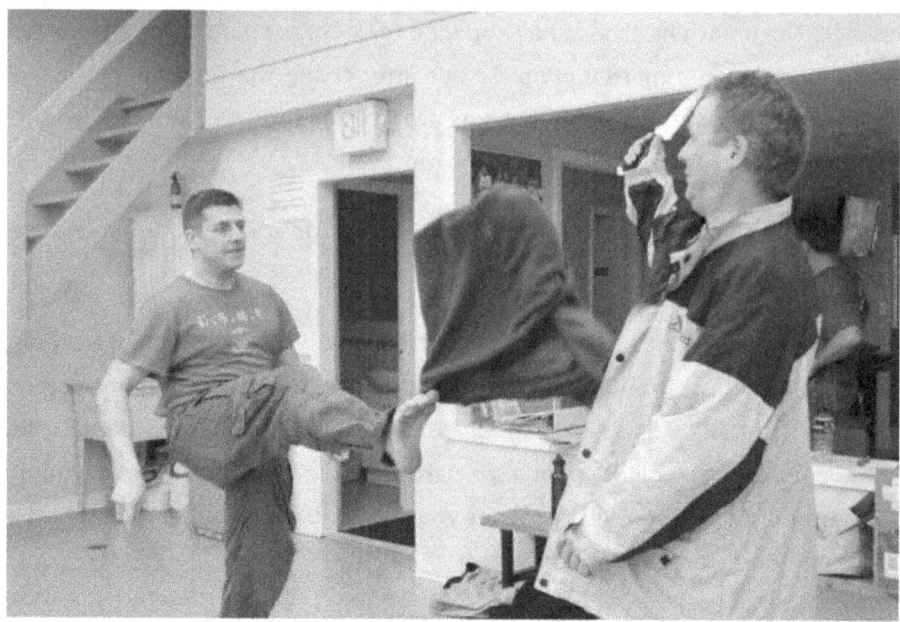

you from all sides. You keep moving, keep breathing and you can get through most things pretty well. I'm CEO of two companies now, I have my own business as Portfolio Manager and I've just taken over the reins of a start up tech company as well.

As a self employed person, how do you manage the stress running your own business?

It's a lot of breathing and relaxation! Because although you don't work 24/7 you do find that you start working as soon as you get up in the morning, especially with the new company. We have team members in Spain, India, Singapore, so there's always somebody awake! There's e-mails, messages, I now have four different chatting apps I never had before, different groups within those, there is always somebody who wants to talk. You have to focus and organise, deal with things quickly when they come in, try not to let them stretch you out. Then when you have a spare five minutes, even if you can't do one of the exercises, you just sit, relax, clean out your tension with the breathing, that's got me through quite a lot.

Finally, do you have any advice for Systema practitioners in general?

The best advice I can give is open yourself up and enjoy doing it. In Konstantin Komarov's book, he talks about the different cycles you go through, you feel like you learn a lot at one stage then you reach another level and you feel like you know nothing. For me, having done other arts in the arts where there were different belts and achievements, well, in Systema we don't have that so you really have to look more at yourself. It was after about three years of training at Toronto, which included periods of frustration, why can't I make this work or that work... one day I was just sitting there before class, just looking around. I said to myself, you know what, I just really love coming here, I don't really care how great I can become at this, I can see myself doing this for the rest of my life. I never had a class in Systema where I didn't leave feeling better than when I went in.

There were plenty of times I didn't want to get into the car and make that 40 minute drive because I felt tired or not in a good mood. But I'd force myself to and within minutes of being in the school, I'd feel better, any tension was gone. Once I started thinking that way, it took a lot of pressure off too. Once that pressure was gone, it allowed me to open myself up more. That's when I noticed my rate of progress really began to improve. A lot of us place limitations or ourselves. It's counter-intuitive to say we shouldn't do that, because you need something, right?

But I think in Systema the main thing you need is just the desire to show up. Because there's enough good people around that if you keep showing up and working on yourself consistently, eventually you will find a way. Have fun with it. All the time, be training, even if it's just breathing, it will make a big difference.

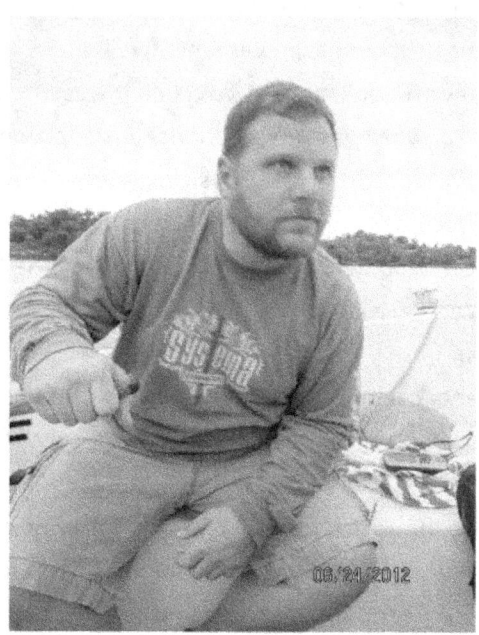

PETE ROGERS

Can you first tell us where you are from and something about your background?

I grew up on the East Coast of Canada in a fishing village, so I was around boats a lot. A lot of family members were fishermen. I had a lot of interest in the outdoors, hunting, fishing, shooting, camping, all that kind of stuff, which naturally led to the military. I was also doing a lot of skateboarding and snowboarding, then got into surfing. I was a snowboard instructor back in the day, I would have been about 17. I was the first in the area and it gave me a good opportunity to learn how to work with people, how to teach and so on, especially as snowboarding was such a new thing back then.

How did you get into the military?

At University I began studying engineering and while doing that I joined the Reserves. After a few years of that I decided to take the plunge and join the regular forces. I was posted to CFB Petawawa as a Combat Engineer.

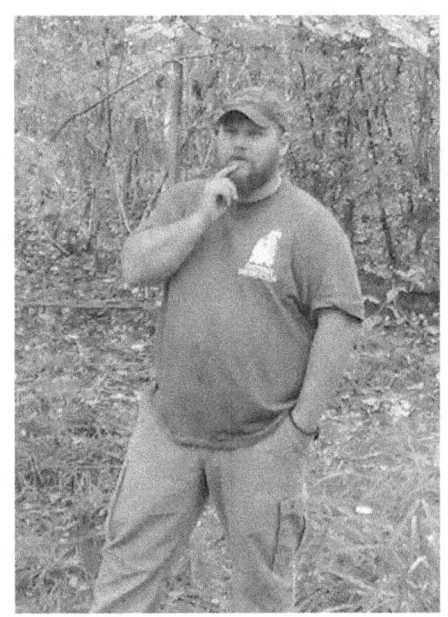

Does your family have a military background?

Well, it's funny, having done research on our family name, Rogers, I found out it was German for *accomplished spearman*! There's been a longstanding tradition of military service in our family. My father served, my grandfather was in World War Two, in fact we've traced it all the way back

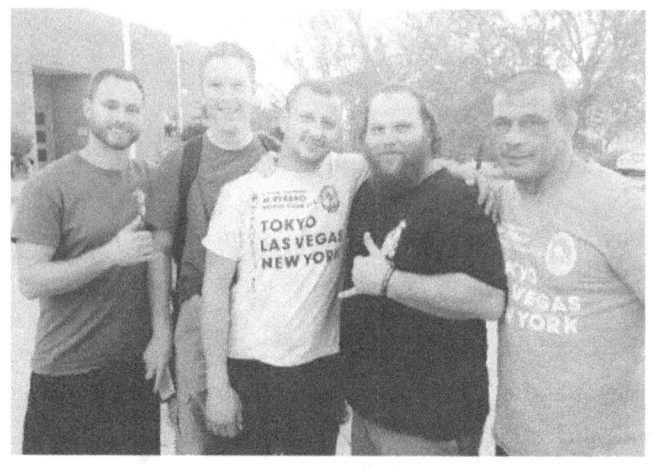

to the Napoleonic Wars. I enjoyed doing that research, seeing how your family came about is fascinating. I guess the breaks and the heartaches they got is what shapes future generations. So yes, there is a family tradition but I also had that interest in the outdoors, plus a sense of patriotism and wanting to serve. But it was funny, because originally I was going to go into the infantry. The gentleman I was speaking to about it was a Combat Engineer and asked me "why the infantry?". I said because I thought that was the main thing, you know, but he said, "Well you should think about the Combat Engineers, you get to do everything the infantry do plus you get to blow stuff up!" (laughs). Of course, what I learned later was, yes you get to blow stuff up but you also have to carry the explosives with you, on foot. And they are a lot heavier than you think, not to mention the picks, shovels and all that stuff!

Where you already training martial arts at the time?

Yes, I started with Uechi-ryu Karate, which is an old Okinawan style with Chinese roots. I also did some Western style kickboxing, this would have been around 1987 and competed in that too. The Karate was a traditional approach, the Senseis were very practical in outlook. Most of them worked in correctional facilities or the fire services. They were very much into breath work too, tough men but good men, I learnt a lot from them. They always encouraged us to look round at other styles too.

What other styles did you get into?

Well there was an American guy who had moved up to Canada after leaving the Marine Corp, he set up a Jujitsu club locally. I remember that to join you had to know someone who was training there and they did background checks on you. That was in the 90s, so I was getting the three things, Karate, Jujitsu and Kickboxing.

And you were competing at that time?

Yes, very much so. It was funny, with the Karate our guys never did so well in Kata competition but they always did very well in the full contact side! I competed on the Canadian Atlantic Kickboxing circuit. My mum was a nurse in the Emergency Department at the local hospital, she was never keen on me doing the fighting, plus riding motorbikes and shooting and the rest (laughs). There were a few times I ended up in the same emergency Room where she was working.

So where did you first hear about Russian martial arts?

Well I grew up with the Rambo culture, you know, fighting against the Russian enemies, so it never came on the radar, not until I was doing military combatives at Petawawa. I was visiting a buddy in Toronto and while there visited Warriors Martial Arts, which was the main martial arts store there back in the day. I noticed some videos he had on Russian military knife fighting, they caught my interest so I bought them. On watching them, I thought the empty hand stuff looked a bit dubious but the knife fighting intrigued me. So that led me to Vladimir and the school in Toronto.

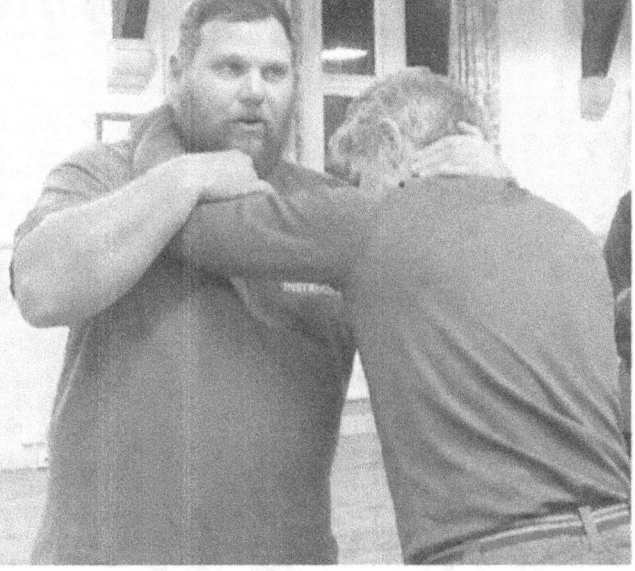

You went along to see him?

Yes. The first time I met Vladimir was at the school. We chatted, I told him about my background and he invited me to join in the class, I thought I'd just hang back and watch at first. After class there was just me and him. I told him I was only really interested in the knife stuff. He said I should try the empty hand too and he could see I was sceptical, so he asked me to come at him. I asked, "What, come at you, or really go at you?" He replied, "You're a soldier, I'm a soldier, treat me like a soldier." So I did! I was a young man at the time, full of beans, so I went at him. Bang, I was down on the mat. I jumped up right away, the only thing my mind could pin it on was that I had slipped! Vladimir smiled and agreed, "Yes, you must have slipped." So I went at him again, the second time, I went down again. I felt zero contact, I'd never have anyone put me down so effortless. At that point I said "Yep, I think I want to start doing this stuff!"

What was the training at the school like back then and how has it developed over the years?

It was pretty rough and tumble back then, everyone was there to learn real stuff.

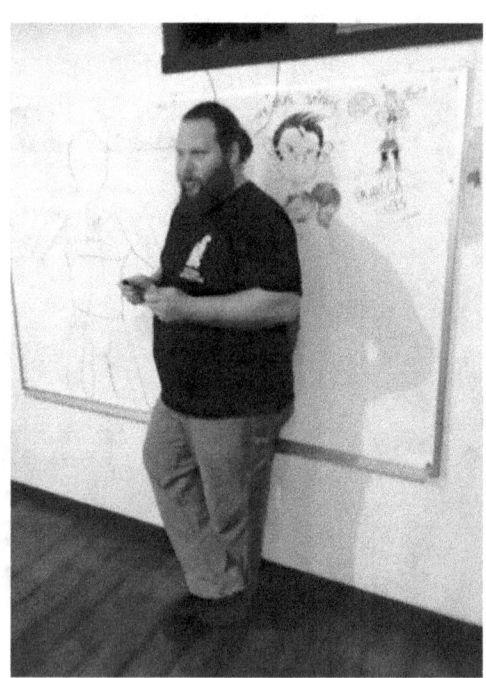

The first couple of weeks I thought people were trying to kill me but after a while I came to realise that they were just being in honest. It's very honest work and challenging. But what really piqued my interest was that it wasn't just physical, there was a very strong mental component, too. It was obvious there was a lot of depth. Seeing how things have progressed over the years, it's a little more refined now. Some might say it's too refined but I don't agree. There is a lot more depth now, more avenues that people can explore.

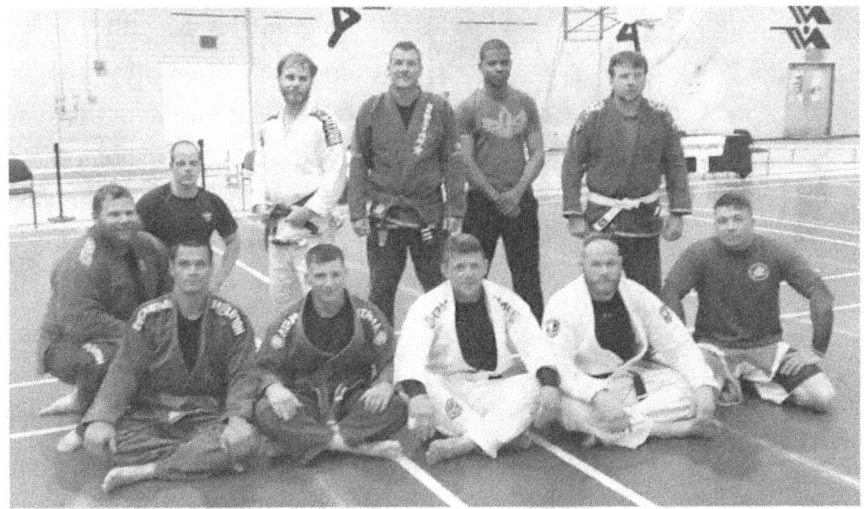

I wanted to pick up on the word "honest" you mentioned there. It seems to me that is a fundamental aspect of Systema and one that people may struggle with?

Yes, it is very important. The first time I really experienced a Systema strike I was very confused. I'd done a lot of body conditioning and Sanchin with the Karate. You could spend hours on Sanchin kata and then it was tested against punches and kicks, so I was used to getting hit. But after that Systema punch, well, that was completely different, I thought "I have to figure this out!"

Was it a surprise to see how soft the work could be as well?

Yes, thought at first I was mainly tuned in to that combatives aspect, hard, honest work. The noticed the subtleties more and more as I went on, to the point I understood that it was the subtleties that defined the art, that made it so effective. It wasn't until I got really serious about my breath work that doors started opening for me and I really started to understand the depth, that was the key in the lock, the breath work.

Were you still in the military at that time and was Systema useful in that regard?

Yes and 100% useful. Here's the thing, if you show a soldier how to make

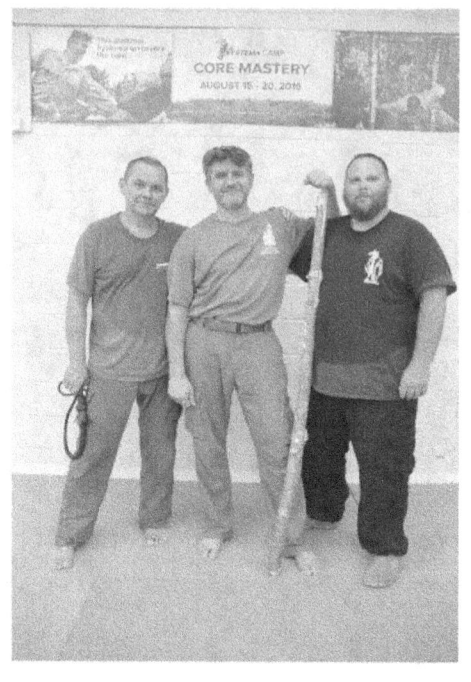

his job even 2% easier, they grasp it. Now people often want to hear how effective it was for this or that, some kind of action scenario but it was the little things that got me. I remember with the breathing, when we did morning runs for PT my running was so much smoother. When I was in, we had the old style Vietnam pot helmets, the heavy ones. Just being aware of holding my head properly helped with that. For me, it's the things that make your day to day life easier, more effective, more enjoyable, I find that very interesting. We had two different states of dress, winter and summer. Summer was sleeves rolled up and that can be from early spring into the fall. Now in Northern Canada there is still snow on the ground in spring! We were in a formation one time in summer dress and it was a very, very crisp day. It was heading towards zero and there was a cold wind coming through too. I started to feel the sting of the cold and I thought back to the whip massage.

As I started to feel the sting I went into the breathing. Then I noticed I was more relaxed, my posture was okay, the cold wasn't such a worry. Looking around I could see the people around me were shivering and these are guys used to the cold. I noticed I wasn't shivering and that's when I really tied it in with the breath work, how effective it was. Such a simple thing but such a big effect. I was a military Combatives Instructor then so I put that into our training immediately. It was a bit of a hard sell at first, there was a lot of testing, shall we say but when they experienced it then attitudes changed. I was always asking Vladimir questions then about the best way to handle this or that, he was always every helpful and patient.

Over here there seems to be a real resistance to anything that helps, when it comes to the services, especially when it is viewed as "soft work".

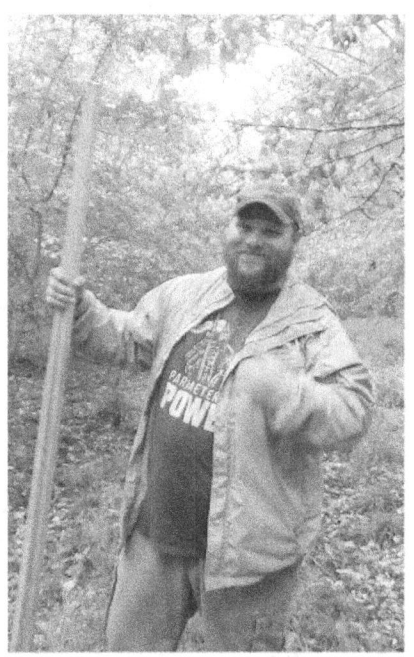

One of the biggest challenges I get with military and police is continuation training. It's getting better now but for quite a period technology was king. More advanced weapons, more tech, more tech based training. What we do focuses more on the individual as the weapons system rather than the equipment. A lot of times there was lip service paid and training was confined to very specific methods, always in blocks. Our approach is more day to day, and it is coming round to that now in some areas. So it was getting guys to keep up the skills. Of course you only have a limited amount of time to get training out to the troops, then they may not be doing it for a while. So how do you get this information across? I came to the realisation that breath work and movement were the two most important things.

Breath work keeps you functional and helps you relax, good posture helps you to move efficiently. And, of course, that plugs into whatever you are doing. But yes, there do seem to be inherent blocks in some organisations where they continue banging against the wall rather than searching for the door. For me Systema provided a door.

Do you think that has something to do with the roots of Systema, way back in the times of the Russian warriors?

I think it's a universal approach throughout many martial cultures. When you are defending your homeland or community you really have to have a commitment to that. People who are used to living a hardy life tend to have a lot more resilience, perhaps. If you have to hike five kilometres to get your daily water, for example, there's a certain mindset and level of resilience that will develop.

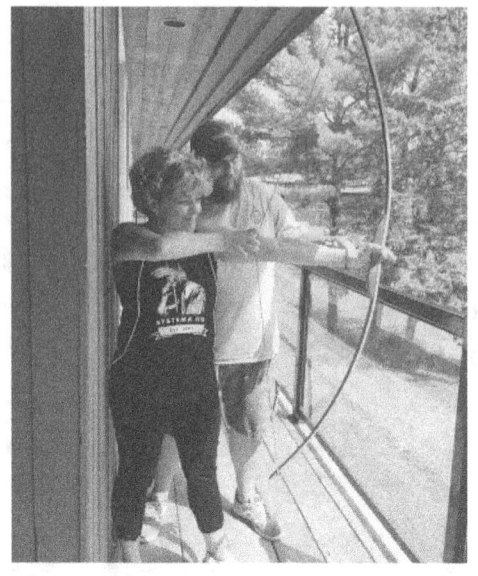

In that respect do you think that System provides a counterpoint to modern, urban life.

For sure. Systema promotes good healthy living. I just came back from British Columbia. The people there are so much more in tune with the land, really resilient, everyone is healthy and smiling. Of course, they have stresses too but they deal with them in a different way. Same back home, making a living from the sea. I remember being five years old out on the boat in rough weather, no lifejacket (laughs). I find that Systema helps build healthy people, it provides a great foundation for being able to deal with stress in all its forms.

I understand you have some experience helping veterans suffering PTSD?

Yes, though I don't use the term "suffering", that's something we are moving away from. It's about stages, in the initial stages it can be quite difficult. It's cyclical as well. For me, personally, that was one of the biggest challenges, that you sometimes cycle back to an earlier stage. I am a Christian, so I have that in my life which helped, plus of course the Systema. I've shared the breath work especially with people and they find it really helps. They've been using things like Yoga for a few years now to help with PTSD but I think the unique thing with Systema is that it has more common principles, it is more applicable. Even if you are confined to a wheelchair, you can practice the breath work. It takes a lot less time to build that connection with the breathing and once there it is a very strong connection. I think in the future we will see a lot more of this approach being utilised in this area.

Speaking of that, do you see that also happening with this growth in interest for natural movement?

Absolutely, there seem to be a value, it develops natural reactions. Or I should say responses, because there is a difference between reaction and response. That's a key thing, Systema is a method to respond rather than react. There's a lot of people in different martial arts, shooting instructors and so on now talking about free movement. But the movement can only be free when the relaxation is there and the mind is free. When you take the core principles of Systema, they are there in all martial arts but it seems to take years in some methods to develop them. We start right off the bat. Think of a Lego set, you are going to make a certain building. You have a picture, you have the pieces, you have instructions, there is a very set procedure in place. Or you might just have a load of Lego pieces and you can make what you like, which is more our way of doing things.

Is that a result of cultural aspects do you think, the power of "tradition"?

One of my favourite statements from Vladimir is "In all things, be human." I think that's the approach that really resonates with people, it transcends culture and background. We all have the same physical make up. Cultural aspects can impose limits, though they may help in getting into certain mindsets. It kind of gives you the key to the code, perhaps. But with Systema, you have that key from Day One. It's about making that connection within yourself, there's your Lego set. You understand that certain blocks in certain ways make shapes and patterns, you have the freedom to explore and experience how these things fit together. What's the old saying "Give a man a fish, feed him for a day, teach a man to fish you feed him for a lifetime."

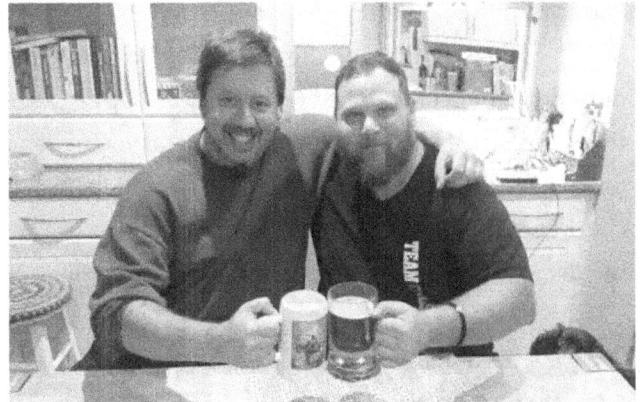

Plus you never see him at weekends! So how did you move into teaching Systema?

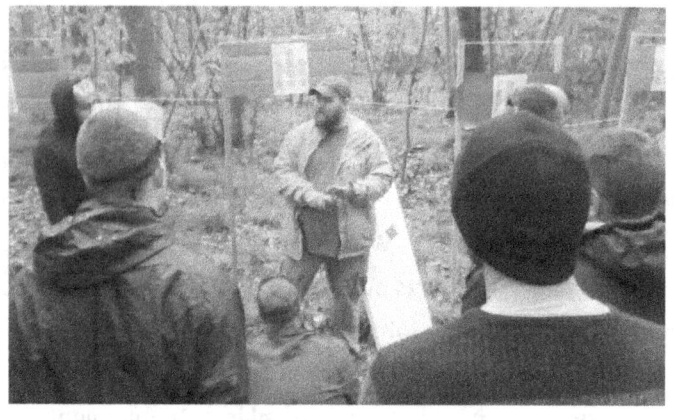

So I was doing those martial arts I mentioned before, plus I also started training in Brazilian Ju Jitsu under Steve Burgess. I find Systema and BJJ really complement each other, more guys round here are starting to see that. There's guys getting great results by putting Systema in their BJJ. I was training military guys and I had a club on base as well. We were doing a mix of things and then I started incorporating the Systema. I kind of snuck it in, I wasn't saying where it was from at first, just getting guys to train certain things. At that time I was also able to bring groups of guys down for private sessions with Vladimir, so there was a lot of learning going on. It helped once people felt things with Vladimir, because at the time I was still working through a way of expressing the work myself.

Did you find that the teaching itself was a learning experience?

There's a tracking teacher I have, David Scott-Doneln, he has a saying "A teacher learns twice." I always loved that, it's true because if you show it, you know it, right? Sometimes you are trying to get something across and people aren't getting it, then of them will say "is it like this?" And then you get a different perspective on how to teach it. This is where humility comes in big time, because if you are stuck on send and you never receive you can miss a lot of good feedback and information from students. So perhaps going back to that cultural thing you mentioned, if the teacher is always right, that's a different mindset and it can take so much more time for learning to occur.

How does Systema affect other aspects of your life? Do you find it working into other activities?

Yes, for sure. Instead of a linear approach I'm finding it's much more about applying principles to anything and everything. For example, I've been doing work with horses lately. There's a guy who in 2015 rode from British Columbia to Newfoundland by horse, he crossed the entire country. It was to raise awareness of veterans and the issues around them. They run a wonderful program for veterans and first responders using equine therapy. I love it so much because what they are doing in effect is Systema with horses. When you see how they are moving these animals, without lead lines or a bit, it's amazing. Horses are so sensitive not to mention always honest! There is so much breath work involved too, plus recognising tension, seeing intent and so on. The tension usually comes from the human too, the horse just reflects it.

The tension we bring into a situation ourselves has a direct effect, right? So you have to find that middle, softer place but still maintain the structure and intent. You have to get rid of the tension so that you can move freely and naturally. Here I was doing this "martial art" and I've found so many different uses for it other than combatives. I use it in shooting, archery, driving, everything really. There's things I'm working on right now, the utilisation of the senses for combat and recovery, for example. Not only for the event but also for the aftermath. This is important for people who are involved in traumatic situations, because it's not always the then and there, it's the afterwards. Some can deal with that but nine times out of ten we see some kind of effect later on. For most of us, dealing with that kind of stuff has its echoes.

And any and every life has its traumatic events, right?

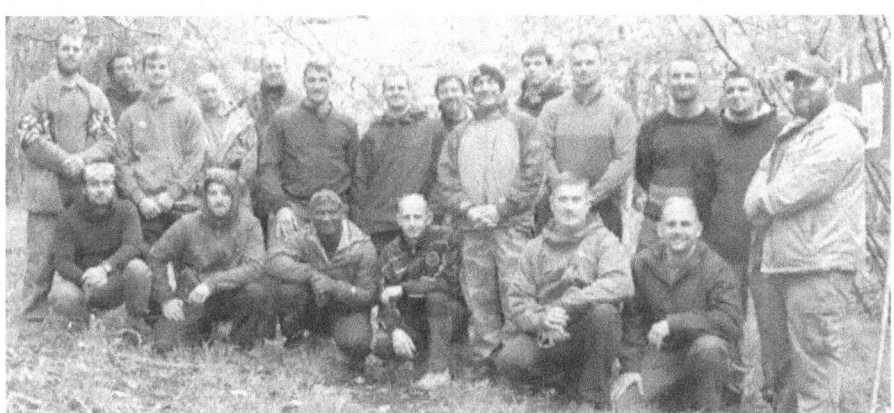

Well someone once told me, some have a shot glass, some have a keg, but everybody fills up. In this day and age, with the technology people tend to be more removed from community. It's strange, because we are more connected in a global sense yet people seem more distant from themselves and each other, we are forgetting how to interact. That also creates issues, too

Going back to the teaching, I heard you are also training guys for MMA now?

Yes, a couple of our guys are now competing in MMA. One had a background as a professional athlete, the other guy is a big guy, a good fighter. It's a joy to train with them, they move well and are intelligent in their approach. There's not much technique-wise I can show, maybe some refinements, but it's mostly about the internal aspects. They've found it really useful, for example in the pre-fight medical they have their blood pressure tested and it has to be below a certain level. One of the guys had quite high pressure, which is normal when people are excited or stressed before as fight. We had a short time to work on it so I took him back into the dressing room and we ran through a breathing drill. The Doc rechecked him and got such a different reading he actually checked his equipment (laughs). It was funny to see, and our man went out and won the fight in 44 seconds.

It was also interesting how that brought a calmness to him pre-fight, there was a definite positive vibe, a good energy. So yes, there's people out there who look upon what we do as weird, esoteric stuff with no place in "real fighting" but you have to know how to breathe! Proper breath work promotes relaxation, that helps identify correct structure and posture, when you have all those elements together you get free movement, whatever you are doing.

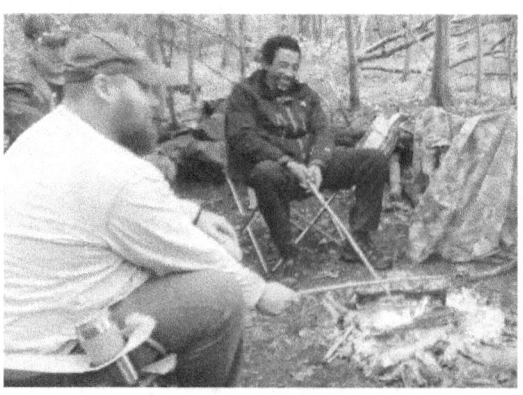

I even did this a few years back with my son's basket ball team at school, I told them I was going to show them "how to slow down time" (laughs). None of the guys were allowed

to shoot at the basket without taking a full breath beforehand. Their score rate went up a huge amount, that was one of the most rewarding experiences, to see how that worked so quickly for them. It allowed them to process all the information much more efficiently and so be more effective in what they were doing.

Do you think this harkens back in a way to our time as hunter-gatherers, where you had to be tuned into the environment? Where, if you check your Iphone, you end up as dinner?

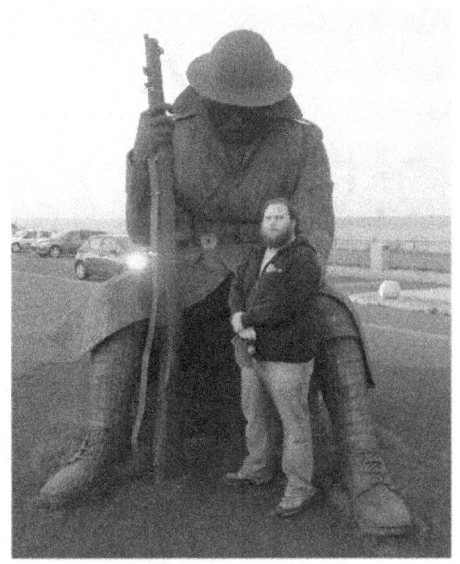

That's so true. How long has it been since us as humans had to worry about being consumed? Now on some parts of the planet that may be true. And I guess even surfing, there have been Great Whites on the East Coast of Canada. I remember my grandfather telling me about a big shark that followed a boat, then rammed it. They recovered the body of one guy, he'd drowned, the other guy was never found. They identified the shark as a Great White through teeth marks in the boat. So there is that, even in our part of the world.

I think I told you about my great fear of snakes? So here it is again, another day-to-day thing where Systema helped. I was mowing my lawn a while back and I saw a big garter snake. Now, we don't have poisonous snakes in Canada, but a lot of places I've been around the world, snakes are deadly. And it's a snake, right! I tensed right up, even though I'm sitting on a ride-on mower that has whirling blades of death. But I'm scared (laughs). So I kicked into the breathing, tuned off the engine and went over to the snake. It took ten minutes but I calmed myself down, I mean the snake was quite relaxed, right? Anyway after ten minutes I was able to pick the snake up. Now I will add this caveat, if you don't know what kind of snake it is, don't handle it! This was definitely a non-venomous snake! But I was able to calm myself down, which kept the snake

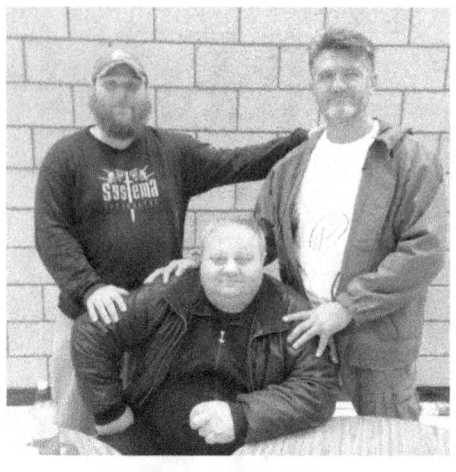 calm and I was able to handle it and move it somewhere safe. So now when I see a snake it's a great opportunity to practice my breathing, to work on my relaxation. I've been doing this stuff since 2001 but every day is learning. You have to be willing to put yourself in beginner shoes, we are always learning, it's an on-going process. Look at Vladimir, for example, his work is so profound yet there is so much humility. There are other instructors I've come across, like Mestre Marcus Soares who brought BJJ to Canada, for example, who have that, but it is so rare.

Do you think that the old way of "teachers-knows-all" is pretty much impossible now?

Yes, because people are more educated these days, everything is on the net. That's a double-edge sword mind you! But that humility is important. In this day and age so many people want to come forward and be an expert on this or that, they tell you they know everything. It's a very closed in attitude. There are core principles for life, whatever you do, when you open yourself up for that it makes a huge difference. Now that is not an easy thing, there is a vulnerability there when you do that. But if you want to talk about humbling experiences, if I think back to some things on a personal level from my time in active zones in the military, there are realities you have to face. It puts things in perspective. With so much stress going on in the world, we need to be more honest with ourselves and put in that humility.

What advice do you have for Systema people?

As a student, don't get frustrated. It can get difficult at times, the approach is a bit of a shift in mindset. It's the little subtleties that really provide the foundation so take it slow, take your time and just enjoy the process. Play more in the grey area rather than the black and white. Allow yourself to make mistakes, that's where you learn. And for all of us, be honest with yourself. Why are you doing this? Why are doing anything? Once your honest you'll get your cornerstone. For Instructors, we are sharing stuff. Keep a sense of humility and wonder. We are privileged that the main teachers are sharing their journeys with us. There are times when you need a bit of structure to get things across, but make sure you are sharing your journey with your students. Don't get frustrated, don't pressure yourself, give yourself the freedom to make mistakes and to be real. Not every demo will be perfect, nor should it be. That's not the real world. You can only share if it's real.

How do you see Systema developing in the future?

For me, I aim to continue on this journey, going into those dark places sometimes and trying to improve my understanding so I can share it with other people. It's been a life-changing thing for me and has helped me in so many ways. It's helped me to relate to people, it's helped me to move better. I have a lot of injuries from my service days, and now I'm carrying a lot of extra weight because of that. Systema has helped me discover a positive mindset and enjoy life a lot better. I'm not saying every day is sunshine and rainbows because there are tough spots, but Systema will help you push through those. When things are going well it also gives you tools to help others around you. We're all in this together, right, none of us gets out alive, so share the good things!

Any last tips or advice for readers?

We don't get to pick when and where our time is done in this planet. There's a lot of examples where you can see that. We do get to pick how we are going to approach things. Rather than focus on getting from A to B focus instead on the journey. Notice things. As you get more information things you thought used to be true may be a bit different, you may find your priorities change. There are times when things need to be black and white, there are times where we can sit in the grey area. Make the best of everyday, be humble and be kind to others. That is a challenge, but if we can share that with other people that is the best, because strong individuals do not survive, strong communities do; strong communities last.

CHINA

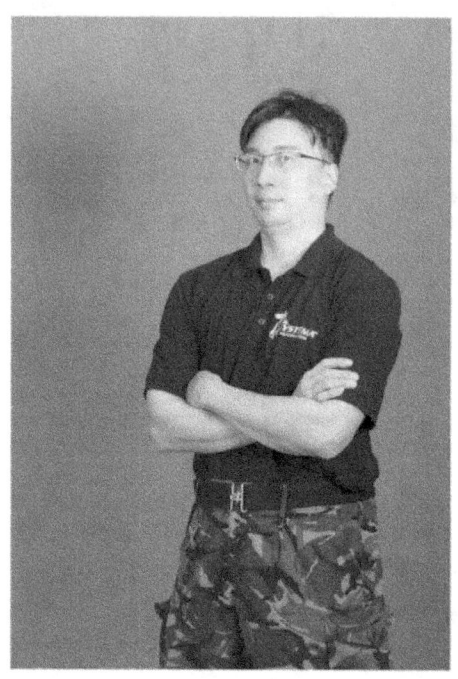

ALI CHUI

Can you first tell us where you are from?

I was born and brought up in Hong Kong. I now regularly hold Systema classes in Hong Kong as a side business and work hard to promote the beauty of Systema in different cities in China, such as Shenzhen, Guangzhou, Zhongshan and Shanghai.

When did you first start training in martial arts?

Like many youngsters, I first started my martial art training during my teenage years under the influence of the Shaw Brothers Kung Fu movies, then, a bit later, Bruce Lee. Why did I start training? Well, to be perfectly honest, I wanted to look cool and be stronger (laughs)! I remember the first martial art I learnt was Wing Chun, that lasted for a few months. Later, I studied Eagle Claw boxing for a couple of years. What I observed was that the training was mostly form (kata) plus a few choreographed sparring sequences. There might also be some conditioning methods, like finger push ups against the wall but it seemed most students were just interested in learning technique. To be fair, I did have some good times after training, going for meals with teacher and classmates, where we talked about historical heroes or usage of skill. From there, I moved into combat sports - mostly Thai boxing - as well as an

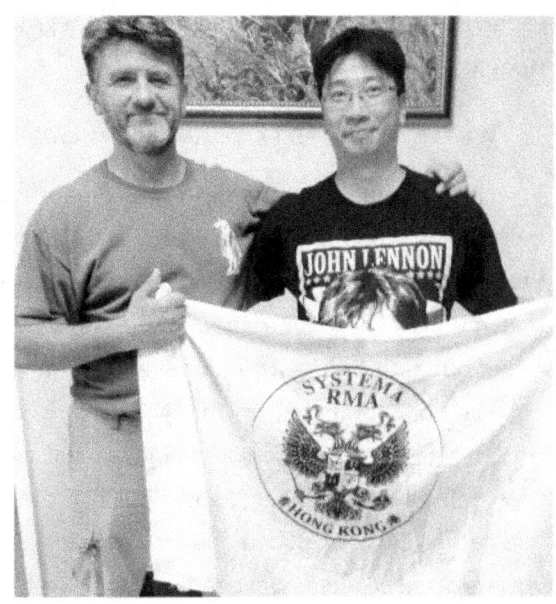

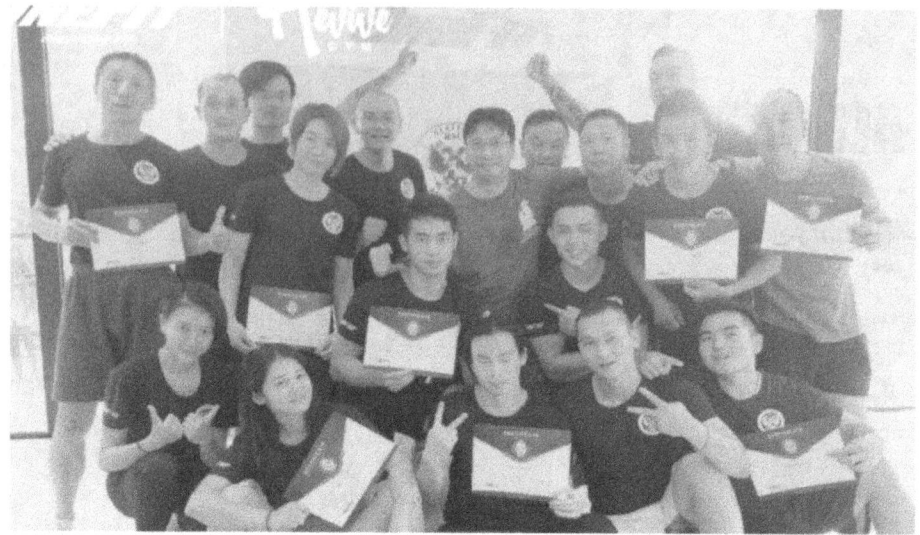

internal Chinese martial art called Yiquan. Considering myself a tourist in martial art world, along with two friends, I also trained in some short courses and workshops in Akido, Judo, BJJ, Kali, Tai Chi and others. So I got the chance to meet masters from lots of different styles.

With the rise of the internet, different styles from Hong Kong and China began to set up friendly sparring gatherings. That was from around the year 2000. I played a role as one of coordinators for those good old times. For sure, I sparred also. I also organized a Capoeria group, I think it was the first one in Hong Kong.

What was your first exposure to Systema?

I first encountered the term "Systema" on a Kung Fu forum, when a friend mentioned that the footwork of Systema was similar to Bagua (one of the Chinese internal martial arts). So I looked it up on Youtube, and I have to say that my first impression about Systema was very sceptical! Later, in 2005, I found out about an instructor called Chi Yip who was supposed to be the first Chinese person that learnt from Mikhail and Vladimir. I decided to visit him to try Systema out in first person. With years of martial art training, it was common to wonder if people swinging like jellyfish can generate so much power. Until you get hit! I was punched and I was convinced. Later on I found out this was what is often called a "wave strike" in the Systema world. Looking into it more, it seemed to me that Systema had everything I wanted - a way to achieve penetrating strikes in a short time, ground tactics, joint locks, pressure point, mass attack, weapons etc, so I decided to settle down!

When did you first meet Mikhail and Vladimir?

It was in 2007, this was the first time I met Mikhail and Vladimir, at the *Masters in Japan* seminar in Tokyo. That workshop I also met Daniel, Edgar, Ryo, Scott, Andy and many more. I certainly had some interesting experiences that weekend, like getting punched and whipped by Mikhail. During the seminar, I joined the queue to get hit by Mikhail. His punch felt like a big 16 kg rocky bowling ball being put into my stomach! That had me bouncing like a ball, I had to burst breath for a minute to ease the tension. For sure, that was far from his full power or I wouldn't be here to write this passage! Another experience with Mikhail was when, after a half day drill of slow push ups, I was feeling very tired and exhausted. He passed-by and gave me some taps with his fist. Ten times or so time downward, then finished with an upward punch...I felt energetic again. This was just one of the weird experiences I had in the beginning stage.

Vladimir was also there that weekend, and I remember that there was a drill to make a big circular movement in order to create tension and make your opponent fall. Once again, people queued up to feel this. Before me I saw some big and muscular guys falling like a tree under a typhoon. When it was my turn, Vladimir used just the first parts of his fingers, not including

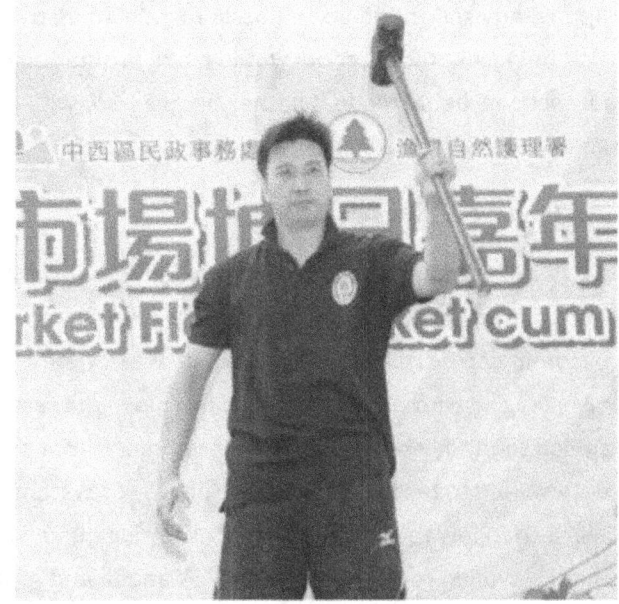

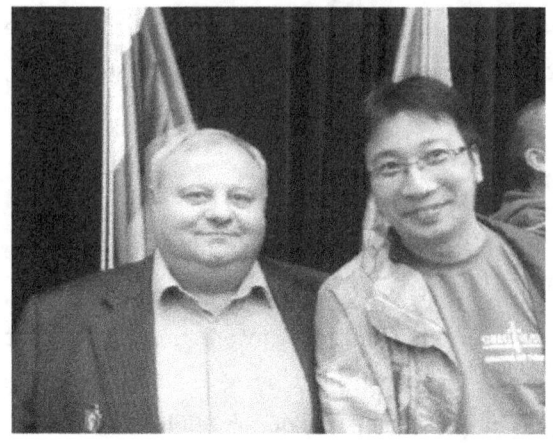

the thumb, to hook my hand and made a small circular movement with his wrist. Tension went through my fingers down to my feet, I jumped and fell like a Japanese anime character given an electric shock! Only difference is that I am real person. (laughs)

How did you begin teaching and when did you set up your own school?

Our Systema RMA Hong Kong group kept on training after some years under Chi Yip, my instructor, until he left Hong Kong for career reasons. So we had a good foundation and with the help of seniors like Eugene and Bhong, we continued our training outdoors in Kowloon Park outdoor and also welcomed Systema fellows from other countries to train with us. Then, in 2012 we moved from the park into my friend's TaeKwondo gym and became more official. At the start, I hadn't really planned to become a Systema instructor but my senior, Bhong, advised me to go to Russia to gain an instructor certificate. We figured that being an official school would make promotion easier and also counter any false claims being made by other people. So, with approval from Moscow HQ, I became a Systema instructor.

How did that feel?

Well, I still remember being at a dinner in Moscow where Ryo San, one of my most respected Japanese big brothers and instructor, congratulated me on becoming an instructor. I replied that I wasn't sure if I was worthy of that, after all having instructor certificate did not make me as good as Martin Wheeler! He smiled tenderly and just said, "Me, neither". That put me at ease and made me determined to teach and share the beauty of Systema. To me, teaching Systema is just to follow the correct path of exploring ourselves and helping others. After that I travelled regularly to Moscow, Canada and Japan for seminars.

How did you find teaching Systema to people from other martial art styles?

With some years of training and teaching, I can observe that people who learn Akido, Tai Chi, Wing Chun or other internal Chinese martial art can benefit most, as Systema drills help them to understand more about tension and relaxation. Systema offers a different angle to observe and decode what they have been doing in their own style, plus our concepts of how to deal with weapons and multiple opponents are very different.

With the help of my martial art friend Ben Cheung, a Wing Chun sifu, I was able to introduce Systema into one of the biggest Hong Kong gyms, the VO2 Fitness Club. Lots of people train there for health, fitness and self defence. My teaching there needed to be less intense, I had to learn to handle people with a little more care, until they're really ready. That's the difference between customers and students.

What, to you, are the defining principles of Systema?

To me, Systema is so much different from what I learnt before. Most martial arts teach you form, kata, a simple set of techniques or skills. Systema is like learning the grammar of a language. Instead of copying the word, phrase, clause or whole text, it shows you how to write your own language of combat through Systema drills. Everyone is unique; maybe physically shorter, tall, fat, slim and mentally bold, cautious, stable or highly mobile. Systema teaches you to work with who you are. Plus, through Systema drills, we constantly change partners, so are always working with people of different size and ability. This teaches our body how to adapt to

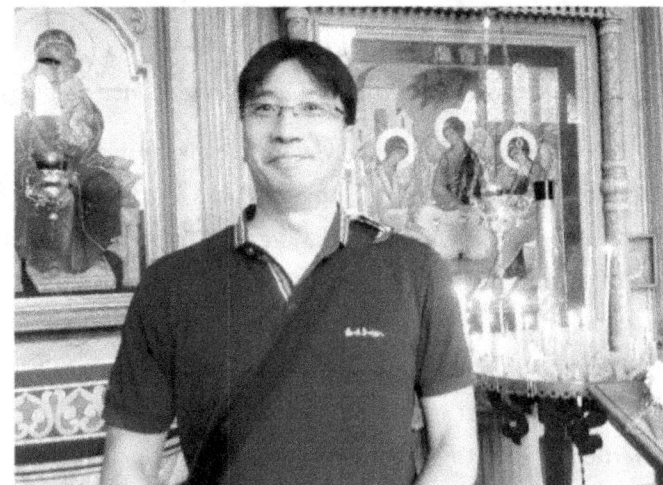

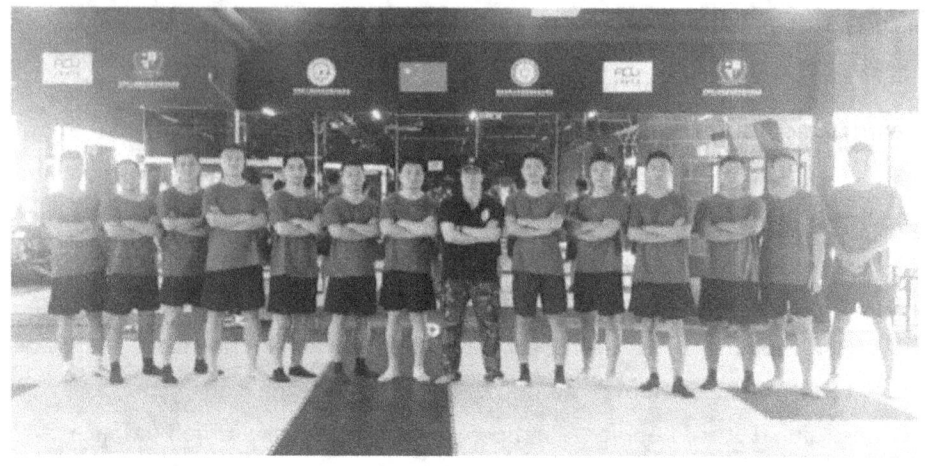

different situations. Hence, I think the grammar of Systema is "Mr. BF", that is Movement, Relaxation, Breathing and Form.

Do you find Systema impacts on your other activities and life in general?

Besides the combat side, I find I often apply Systema in daily life. For example, when there is an argument, you can move away from a person's line of attack and redirect them, instead of trying to crush them. So instead of saying "I don't agree with you," try saying "I agree with your viewpoint," follow his tension and redirect. Don't block, redirect as Systema teaches. Of course, this is a very simple application of Systema principles in a non-physical situation, there are many other examples.

Have your goals and priorities changed since you began training?

My training goals initially were to roll smoothly on hard flooring, to achieve a penetrating punch and to do joint locks and takedowns effortlessly. I managed to achieve those within my first year of training. Nowadays, my training goal is to be a good person to have a healthy life and also have some combat skill.

Mentally, I work to be a good person through using "Mr BF" so as to have better personal relationships with others, the society or the universe in general! Surely, it is better to avoid conflict in the first place if you can. Still, Systema is a martial art, like the function of the knife is to cut. The combat side of Systema is still my concern, how to protect yourself and your family when needed.

Physically, my priorities are much more now on how to tackle knife attack and work against multiple opponents, as these are the most dangerous street situations. That aside, to me, Systema is now a complete attitude of lifestyle, wider than just the combat side.

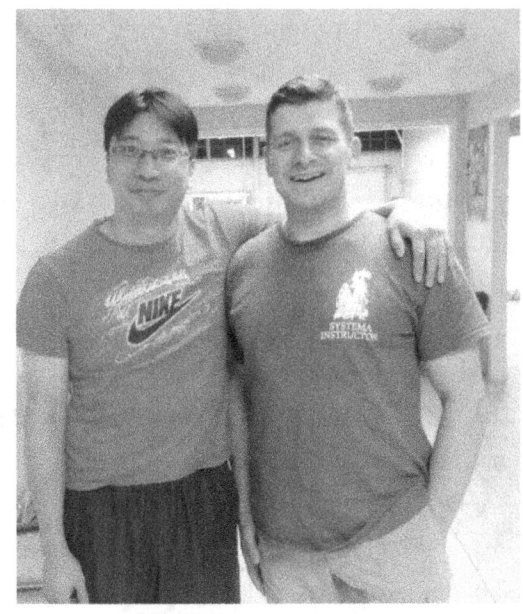

How many classes are you teaching now?

I train with students outdoors in the park on a Wednesday and indoors every Saturday at the Momentum Fighting gym (owned by my Muay Thai friend, Alfred Kwong). Every Thursday and Friday night, I teach Systema classes at the VO2 Fitness Club.

What do you think is the best way to approach learning Systema?

Stay humble and calm, mutual helping, relax and observe your body inside. Don't rush, be patient. No ego, no arrogance, no pride, less emotion.

Do you have any advice to instructors on how to structure their sessions?

First and the foremost, the most important thing is to create a relaxed atmosphere, I usually use square breathing with walking for students. Don't skip that before any technical aspect or application as it creates a little time for the body and mind to be ready. Keep observing all the students during the session. If you find they are struggling, the instructor can stop and get students to go back to some basic drill, like wall squats for example. This was one little trick I observed in the Toronto HQ lessons with Vladimir.

When you go somewhere new and teach a group of people, how do you organize the training?

Just to share some things from when I go teaching in China, I usually start by saying "Every martial art is good and I am here to offer you something new," so as not to create conflict. Usually I will first show some effect of Systema teaching since the power generating way of Systema is so weird and different from the general. After the "What is Systema" bit, I then come back to "How" and "Why"? Taking the Systema punch as example, I let them feel a strike first before asking them to do pushups. Of course, you have to be careful not to hurt students and also not to fill up your own ego. I've seen people punching really hard and hurting students, using the excuse that "you should be prepared". That is not a good approach with new people, that approach is more about the instructor's ego.

I've taught many times seminars surrounded by fitness coaches and instructors from other martial arts. Reaction is always positive, I find if they are shown the process and progression, they become much more patient when it comes to breathing drills, for example. But it is a fine balance. Mikhail once said a while back, "Don't hide your skill too much, even if you are being nice." I find that good metaphors always help teaching students. For example, punching as if you are eating with a knife and fork. We can go one step further; for example using technical terms of computing as metaphors if your students are IT people to help get your point across.

What other interests do you have outside of Systema?

Apart from Systema, I also enjoy rowing, HEMA weapon sparring, reading and watching movies. Currently, I am adviser for International Wing Chun Association, Vice-chairman of Hong Kong Chong Yi Association (Yiquan), Promotor of Utimate Kombat Alliance (weapon sparring). Also, I was the

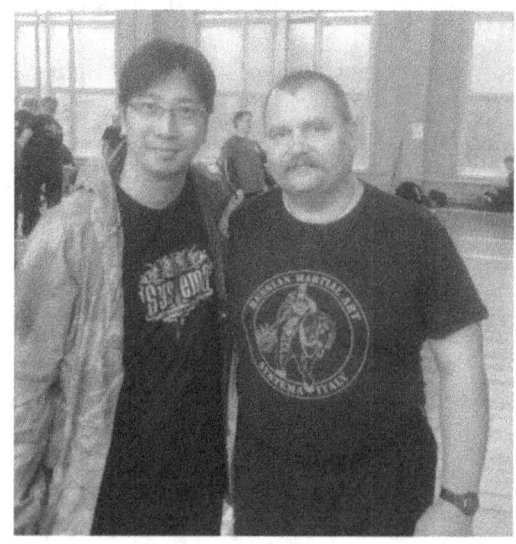

founder of Capoeira Beribarzu Hong Kong and used to be Coach of the City university Rowing team.

How do you see Systema developing in the future?

In the future, I wish more people will learn and enjoy Systema and I hope to meet more people from the Systema world. To clarify some misunderstanding on Systema, no one will force you to become an Orthodox Christian or keep you from "secret techniques" if you do not. I can see lots of senior students who are already good fighters. This is fine but it is good to go Moscow, to taste what is the "internal work" of Systema. Without internal work, you can still be a good fighter but internal work offers some smart ways of power generation and teaches you how to be very precise in your work.

My observation is that Systema may not fit everyone. Some people come but may not stay for too long, because Systema is not so much about one-on-one competition. Surely, Systema is more about survival than competition and this is fine. Of course, breathing, strikes, movement drills, aerobic exercise of Systema, are all starting to gain some interest from the MMA world. So you can observe now how some other people "borrow" a Systema drill, give it a new name, such as "xyz challenge" or combine some Systema drills together to make a "new system" for money and marketing. Of course you can't use "intellectual property rights" on movement. But maybe we can do more to let the general public know what we are doing through marketing. If we can spread understanding of what Systema is really about, I'm sure more people would come into it.

Any last words of advice for the reader?

Nothing more to say, just start training, have fun and I hope to see you some day!

SYSTEMA VOICES

GERMANY

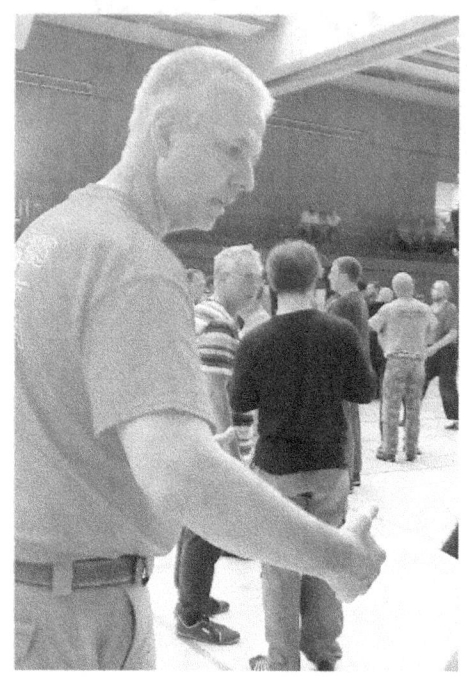

NORBERT TANNERT

Could you please first tell us something about your background

I was born and grew up in Krefeld, about 100km from Bonn. At school I was very interested in swimming, I competed in the German Championships. I was training for the Olympics in 1980, which were unfortunately cancelled due to politics at the time. In that year I joined the police and have been a police officer ever since. I served 22 years within Special Forces, then in 2011 came back to Bonn and am now Commander of the Mid Town Police Office here.

So was a lot of your police work quite specialised?

Yes, in my time with Special Forces I visited a lot of countries, including England. We have good contact with SO19, for example. I travelled all over Europe, we've also had a team from Ireland come to visit us for an exchange. I also travelled to the USA to work with the LA Sheriff's Dept, also the SWAT teams in Oklahoma. So quite a lot of travel!

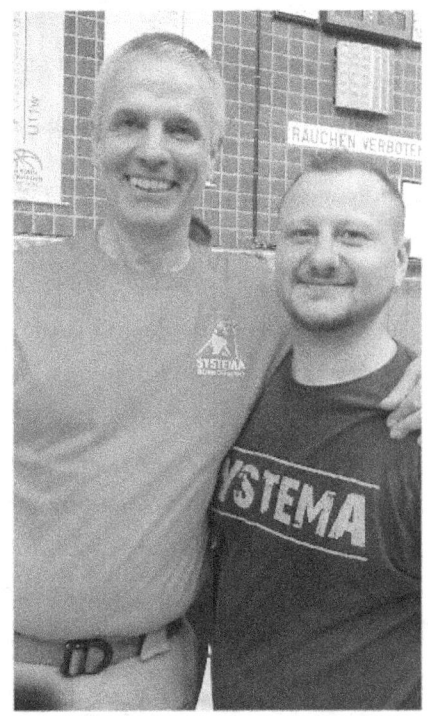

Do you find that policing varies around the world or is it more similar, based on current threats?

When I was doing the Special Forces trips I found the work was very similar. You always had the feeling that when you went somewhere to visit another group, it was just the same as your own people (laughs). The talk, the humour, it is all very much the same around the

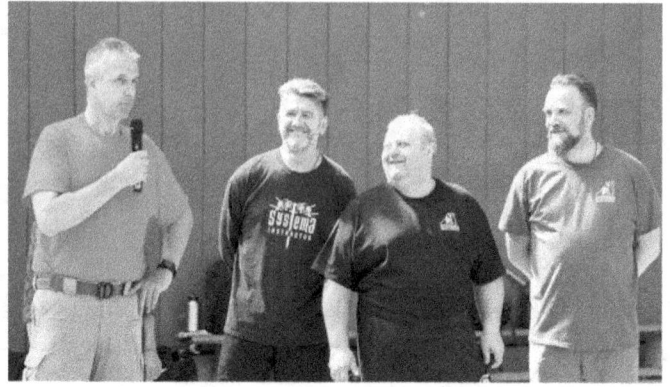

world! I guess the big difference now is that the ordinary, front line officers are the ones facing the big threats. They are the ones who have to deal with a terrorist attack, for example. It has changed a lot since Paris and we don't know where things will go at the moment. It is an unsettled time right now. Yet when I first started Systema, that was a time when things seemed to be changing for the better

True. I guess our generation grew up in the Cold War, under the perceived threat of nuclear attack. It changed for a while but now that tension seems to be back again?

That's it, it's not exactly the Cold War again now but it is uncertain. Everything is now called into question.

When did you first get interested in martial arts?

It was in 1980, when I joined the police. I started with Ju-jitsu and got a dan grade there. However, I was finding it difficult to apply on the street, so I began looking at other things. I trained in Bujinkan Ninjitsu for 12 years under Hatsumi. But after a while I began to have some differences with my teacher at the time and it was unpleasant how we got treated. I was working with the Special Forces then and I saw that the reality was not what was being trained for. But, of course, if you questioned what was being shown, that was not at all appreciated. It got so bad I was thinking about quitting martial arts as a whole, I was very disappointed with many aspects of it. If there is an unbalance between what is taught and what is done, it is not healthy, even if you take out the question of reality, just on a personal basis.

And was this when you first saw Systema?

Yes, I friend of mine brought in a video of Vladimir, his first knife video I think it was. He played it when we trained together, we were just training in our own group then. I watched it and said, "This is crap, I don't like it, this will never work!" (laughs). But my friends were interested and said we should check it out. At the time there was a guy in Augsburg, Andreas, who had been training Systema already, I was still not that keen but my friends were very insistent that it was good stuff! At the end of the day I said okay, I'll go to Toronto and check it out. So I wrote to Vladimir, not expecting any answer but I got a reply within days. It was a very welcoming letter, so I flew over for three weeks. And, in a way it was very awful for me!

Because it neutralised everything you had done before?

Totally! I couldn't do anything! Nothing! Almost 20 years of training and I struggled with the exercises, I couldn't move correctly, couldn't roll correctly, I felt I couldn't do anything! But that showed me Systema's worth and from then on I really wanted to get into it.

Did you also find that although you were not effective against the Toronto guys, it was a positive experience, rather than being "beaten"?

Exactly. This was a total difference to what I had experienced before. Vladimir moved with ease and dealt with everything with no aggression, that's what impressed me the most. That I couldn't do it was annoying for me but no-one judged me on that. At the end of the three weeks it was clear that what I had done before was of hardly any use, so I threw it away

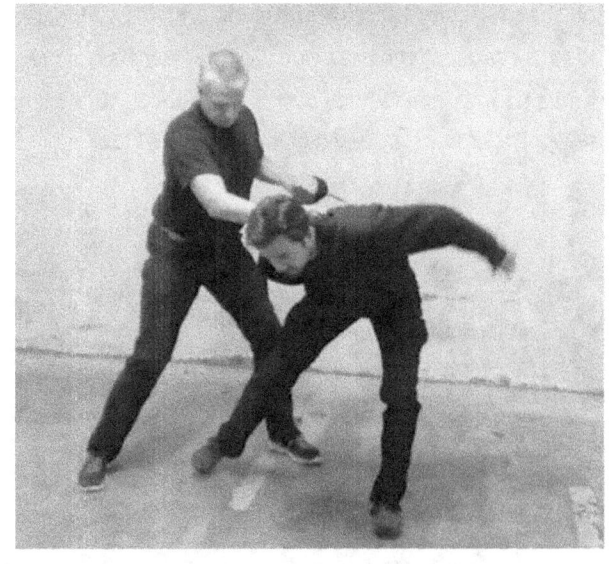

completely. Even the books and t-shirts I had from before, I threw it all away, I wanted to start completely from new.

It was a complete break?

Yes, for me I couldn't do it in bits, it had to be this way.

What have been the biggest benefits for you in training Systema, both professionally and personally?

Well, it changed my whole opinion of martial arts. It showed that the main focus of martial arts is not being stiff, aggressive and dominating but to be relaxed, mentally and physically. This, to me, brings the biggest benefits. You get calmer, which is not a bad thing when you are working with Special Forces! You learn to deal with stress on all levels, not just combat wise but in life in general. But especially when it comes to combat.

I always find it funny that people think Special Forces get all sorts of secret, advanced hand-to-hand training - in fact this doesn't happen. You get to train maybe once a month and everybody hates it (laughs). Of course everyone is able to hit someone or get them on the ground to restrain them, but there are so many other demands when it comes to operations and training, that the hand-to hand work is far down the list. I sometimes see advertising about this or that "special forces" methods and it is all wrong. This is where Systema is ideal because it teaches people how to relax, how to deal with threats in a calm and serious way. But also, it is for everyone, anyone can do it, not just Special Forces!

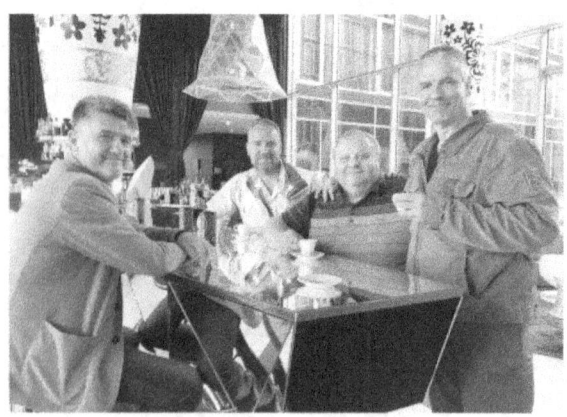

Do you think Systema is something that goes back much further than modern military use?

Of course. If you look at the movements and think about how a sword is used, you can see where it comes from. So it seems that some people in the past knew things that were quite good! Remember that people in those days were fighting for their lives, that 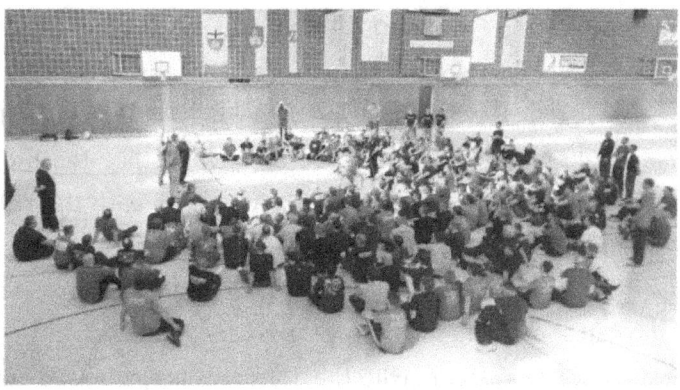 changes things totally. The one who is the calmest in this situation will win, the total opposite of how some arts are advertised today. Now, in many places they teach people to really be over aggressive, which means they lose awareness of many things. It's a shame that people think that is the correct way, they even injure themselves in the training.

Speaking of swords there is a lot of interest in historical fighting in the UK at the moment, do you have that here?

There is a big scene in Germany for this, in different ways. Some are more about re-enactment, others go really hard at it with real, blunted weapons. They have the books of Durer, he did some artwork on sword fighting and unarmed fighting in Renaissance times which the people now try to translate into movements. The difficulty is in getting movement from a still image, you can maybe miss the part in-between each movement. The pictures are also, perhaps suggestions, so it is fun but it's not necessarily the real thing.

I am very much into history but not so much into work with historical weapons, because I think if you train in Systema for a while and see how it approaches weapons, you will find that it is quite different from much of the re-enactment work.

When and how did you start teaching Systema?

Teaching was never a main idea for me. We had a club running when we were doing the Eastern arts and when we changed over, we taught because we had to, no one else was there! It was hard at the start, we had just made the first trip to Moscow in 2002 , we got some ideas of what to work on. Mikhail gave us a good amount of work on the basics, particularly breathing. So that's what we taught when we came back. The same today, really, every time we go and train with the masters, we bring what they teach us back to show our people. As well as my class I'm still working with the police guys, which is a different emphasis. But they have been very receptive to it. I found the same with teaching the Special Forces guys. I didn't call it Systema at first, I just showed some things and they were very appreciative.

Same now, I work with the normal police, we have quite a high crime rate here. There's a lot of violence against policemen, for example, so I started to work with them, on a voluntary basis and it is working very well. The street officers benefit from it, they changed their behaviour while on patrol which has been helpful. Plus of course, we train things like restraint work and similar. It gives the officers self confidence, which makes then more relaxed with people. Then they are not responding from a place of fear, it helps to keep situations calm.

What is your main emphasis when teaching?

For me teaching is about showing things that I know are practical, and with my work I know what is practical!! Just last week I had to take a guy to the ground (laughs). So Systema has changed my opinion on many things and how they work. I'm always looking to the practical side of things and that's my main focus with our club. Then, on the other side, we all have to deal with stress, whatever our job is and I think Systema is the peak of learning to manage your stress. If you can

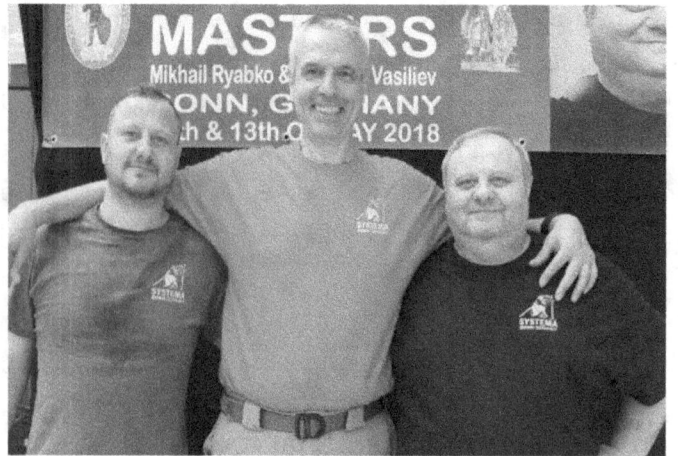

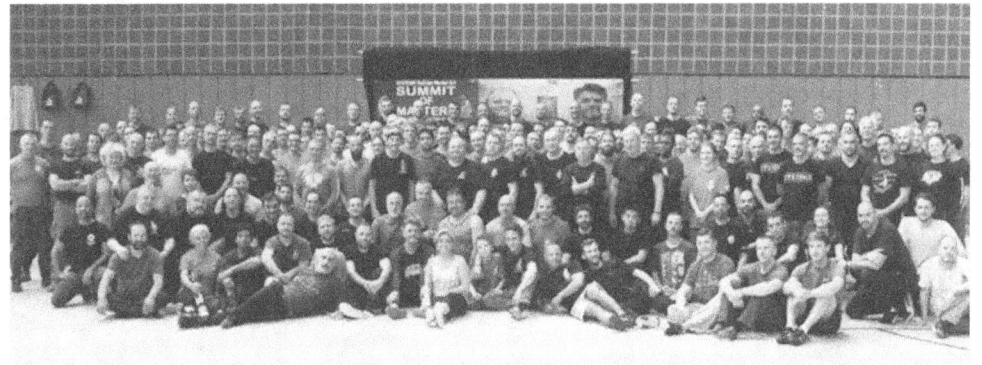

control your stress in a potentially dangerous situation, that's the key. It's not physical, it's that psychological control.

What Systema plans do you have for the future?

I've not done so much outside of my police work as there are many Systema teachers around now, there's no need for me! (laughs). But what I usually do, outside of the police, is travel to teach people I know. So I am going to France soon, also Austria, that's always fun. If friends ask, I go, I don't really teach as a business. I think to do that you need to be very alert as to what is going on, to keep a healthy balance between money and the teaching. For me, I am in the position to help friends, I have a lot of fun but if people I don't know ask then I am not so keen.

Do you have any last thoughts to finish on?

I think, looking back, there were some difficult times with my old style. There have also been critics about Mikhail And Vladimir in the past, but at the end of the day I'm very thankful that I've found them and that I have had a chance to learn from them. They both have made a lot of effort to teach someone who must have been totally annoying (laughs). I still feel very thankful about that, so this is it, these are the guys to learn from!

SYSTEMA VOICES

JAPAN

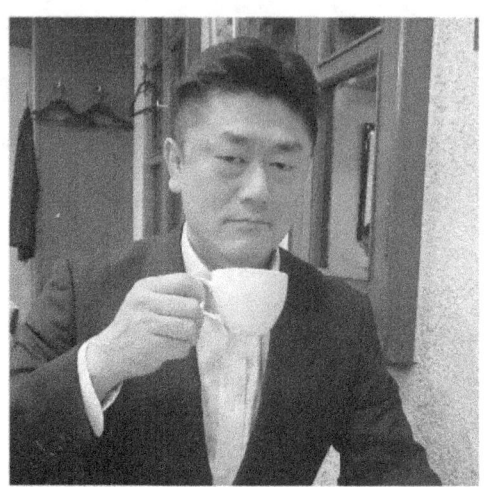

RYO ONISHI

Could you first tell us where you are from?

Yes, I am from Osaka in Japan and my occupation is as a localisation specialist and translator

How did you get into martial arts training and when did you first see Systema?

My first martial arts experience was in Japanese arts, due to a friends's recommendation and the training was painful! Later, it was my Japanese martial art teacher who introduced Systema to me, live first, then video.

What were your first impressions?

I couldn't really figure out what it was, I hadn't even heard of it before. But my teacher thought it was good idea and he began showing us Systema exercises.

When did you first meet Vladimir and Mikhail and how did you find the training?

It was at a seminar in the UK, then later I trained with them at Systema HQ when I became an Instructor. The training was very different, it was like nothing I had ever seen or done. It was so free.

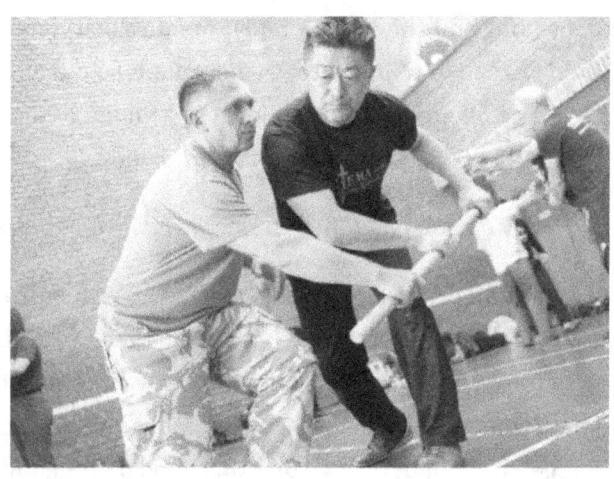

Have you found that Systema has impacted on your life in general?

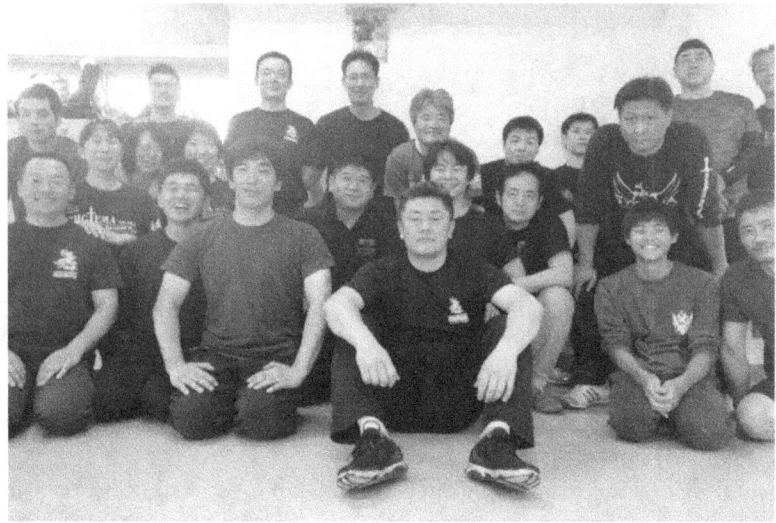

Definitely, because I find that good Systema concepts work anywhere, anytime! I am healthier and a little better person because of it. It has affected my perception deeply. I also find that the training is changing all the time.

How did you find it when you began teaching?

At first I was trying to teach Systema in the Japanese martial arts way and I didn't get far! I was struggling, I think. I was always looking for more exercises. But when I started to spend more time with the masters, that changed gradually and naturally.

I also began to see that the training encompassed everything about human behaviour and the human body, mental health as well as physical health. So then instead of trying to teach individuals so much, I worked instead to control the atmosphere and tension level as a whole in the gym. I aim to relax people so that they will have different point of view.

How do you feel that Systema has developed over the years?

I think that when Mikhail started to emphasize more internal aspects of training, the work started to go deeper. When you spend more and more time with him, you will catch the state/presence and this will help you to feel the key elements until it clicks for you. Make the most of it. Don't try too much to intellectually understand something you didn't know . If it's completely new to you, you will have no means to judge the stuff anyway so take it as it comes... so that even if it's vague to you, you still have everything, you have the experience. When you truly understand something, everything else will fall into place.

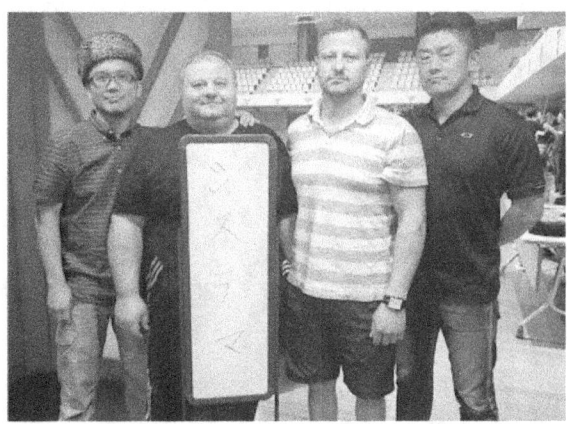

As your training goes on in Systema, do you appreciate more the depths of training?

Yup. If we can get better without getting stronger, faster or tougher, we are getting better in Systema, in my opinion. So as a result, almost as a side affect, you will become stronger, faster and tougher. To me Systema is a way of life. I hope I can go deeper with it and become slightly better person.

Lastly is there anything you would like to add for our readers? Any advice or thoughts?

Systema gives different perceptions and realizations. Spend as much time with the masters as possible, whenever possible, wherever possible. It's okay even if you are not in the conversations, stay close in the distance, you can listen to them and feel their presence/state. By doing that your state will get affected and this will help you to perform better, until it wears off. During this time, you will peek into the level of work that you couldn't do it before and realize the importance of your internal state, rather than relying on techniques, power, speed, and even precision.

And then, in practice, instead of trying to do something to the opponents, try to move in such a way that you improve your state in all levels. Try to move in such way that after the movements you are cleaner than before(in tension). Dealing with the opponents should be a side affect of that choice. I hope you will find what you are looking for!

PERU

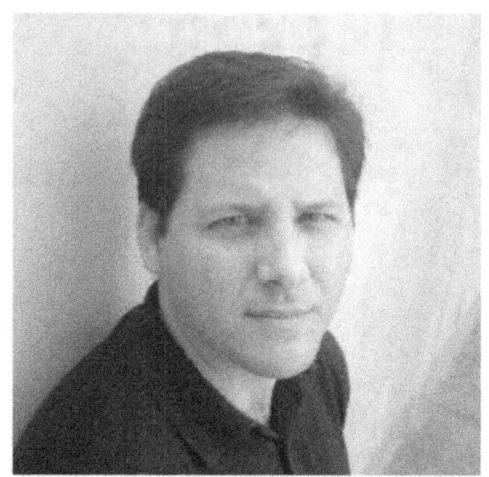

BRATZO BARRENA

Could you first tell us something about yourself?

My name is Bratzo Barrena, I was born in Lima, Peru, on October 19th, 1970. I'm married with two daughters. Currently I work as a Systema Instructor at my school Systema Ruso Combate Funcional, in Lima.

When did you first start training in martial arts?

As with most people, I started training martial arts for self-defense purposes. My parents, enrolled me in a Karate school when I was around 7 years old. I trained for a couple of years. At age 13 or 14, I also trained Taekwondo for a while. In 1993, I started training Aikido, I became a shodan (black belt) in 1997. In 2001 I moved to New York and trained at the New York Aikikai for a few months. Then I moved to Miami, where I trained and taught in a couple of Aikido schools until I opened my own Aikido school. I always considered Aikido as incomplete, that's why while training/teaching Aikido, I also trained BJJ and Muay Thai, as a complement, to add in what I considered Aikido was lacking.

When did you first see Systema and what were your impressions?

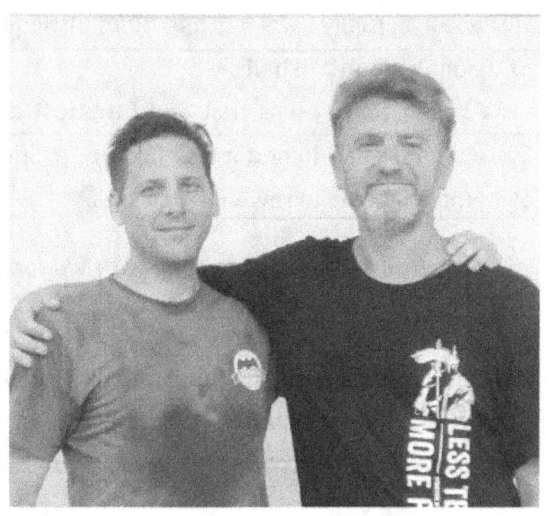

In Miami, in 2005, I was watching Aikido videos on the web, while suddenly, an Aikido Journal's video popped up presenting this guy and his students dressed in camo, performing techniques that looked fake, rehearsed and ineffective. I knew Aikido

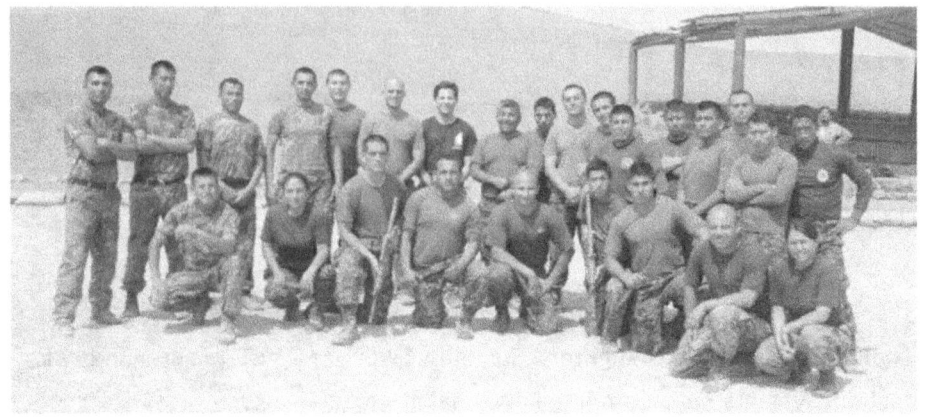

videos looked fake, but this guy's video was even worse! The guy in this video was Vladimir Vasiliev. For some reason, every time I was watching Aikido videos, these guys in camo popped up. Now, this bulky guy punching people standing in a row... okay, this caught my eye. I didn't understand why these soft, slow punches seemed to hurt so much. Are their reactions real? Are they faking it? If their reactions were real, it would be awesome, but are they? This bulky guy was Mikhail Ryabko.

I kept watching Vladimir's and Mikhail's videos as they popped up, and as I saw them, began to see that their "techniques", even though at first glimpse they seemed fake and ineffective, were actually the most impressive demonstration of bio-mechanics, timing, and spontaneous movement... I knew I didn't completely understand what they were doing, but now it didn't look silly at all, actually I was getting quite intrigued by the subtlety and efficiency of Vladimir's and Mikhail's work.

At that time, I was first and foremost an Aikidoka, but decided to give Systema a try and joined a training group. Soon, I started implementing some Systema concepts in my Aikido classes.

From there you went to train with Vladimir?

Yes. Well, back in Peru, I continued teaching Aikido, but a good friend of mine and I were becoming more and more interested in Systema. He contacted Nelson Wagner, an Instructor from Brazil, and we organized the first Systema seminar in Lima, Peru. After this seminar, we knew we would dedicate ourselves exclusively to training Systema. Soon after, we contacted Systema Headquarters in Toronto, Canada, and our direct relationship with Vladimir's school began. We opened the first Systema academy in Peru. We would regularly organize training seminars in Lima, inviting international instructors such as Nelson, Frank Arias and Maxim Franz. In 2013, I opened my school Systema Ruso Combate Funcional.

What was it that drew you in to Systema?

I found in Systema everything I was looking for... and much more. Systema is a complete self-defense martial art, it covers all aspects of a confrontation: physical, mental, and emotional. I was impressed by its subtlety, power, and effectiveness, derived from relaxation, movement, and limitless spontaneity. Explaining Systema to a non-practitioner, I may dare say, is an impossible task; mere words cannot describe its depth. You must feel it to understand it.

Do you find that people can struggle with it at first, as it is so different?

In the beginning, its training methodology is difficult to understand. In martial arts people are used to training following a very strict set of movements or techniques that one must repeat continuously to develop "muscle memory", until they become reflex reactions. But Systema is very different. It has no pre-established movements or syllabus of techniques that you must memorize. Freedom of movement is the most important aspect, this is why training is based on discovering all the possibilities of movement your body has. This methodology develops what I call "muscle intelligence" and your reactions become spontaneous, free, and unlimited.

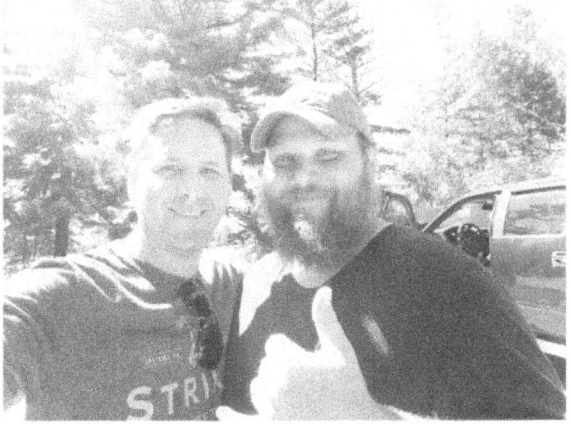

We must be careful, there is a subtle difference between "there are no

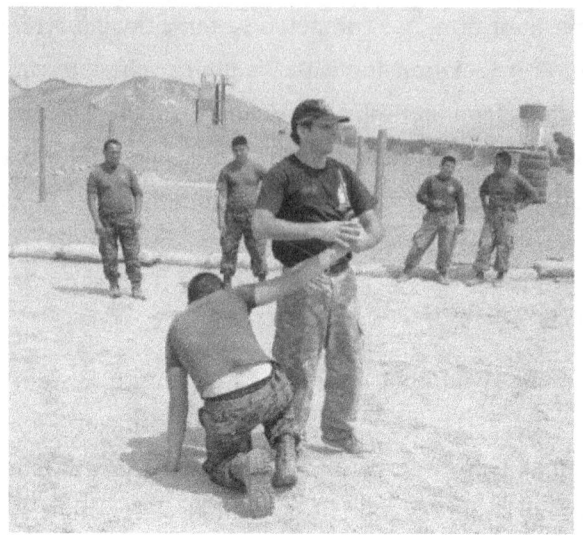

techniques" and "there is no technique" in Systema. Every single movement or posture we are in utilizes biomechanics; but not all movement, posture or form is biomechanically efficient. In this sense, in Systema there are no techniques if we refer to memorizing a syllabus of pre-established movements, but it does have technique if we refer to developing the ability of efficiently using your body bio-mechanics.

And, of course, there is the huge emphasis on breathing too.

Breathing training in Systema also made a deep impression on me. It was much more than just filling up my lungs with air. In Systema, breathing is a tool to improve your physical performance, tune your mental awareness, and balance your psyche. And I'm not talking about developing ki, chi or any other mystical force, like some other martial arts may claim. Systema has a down-to earth approach to breathing. Through a series of practical and simple drills, Systema breathing teaches how the flow (or lack of) of oxygen into the body has an impressive effect on one's overall performance, and how you can regulate your breathing to reduce fatigue, mitigate and recover from pain, and calm your emotions to overcome stressful situations; and, most important, this is an ability that will transcend into every facet of your daily life.

You mentioned self defence as a reason to begin training earlier, how do you classify "self defence"?

Most martial arts and combat sports claim to be designed for self-defense, but that's not an accurate statement. This misconception comes from misunderstanding what self-defense really is. Most people agree that fighting in a tournament or competition is not self-defense, it is a duel. But they might consider any "street fight" as self-defense, they are wrong, most street fights are also duels.

Systema helped me understand that there is one key difference between a duel and a self-defense confrontation. To explain it in a simple way, in a duel two (or more) people want to dominate the other, they want to "win"; while in self-defense, one person (or more) wants to hurt someone, and this someone doesn't want to get hurt, this person wants to survive. This subtle difference changes completely the dynamics of a confrontation. To understand Systema, its training methodology, concepts, application, effectiveness and goals, it's necessary to understand this difference. Once you understand what self-defense really is, you also understand that your fighting capabilities shouldn't be restricted by techniques or specialization.

And Systema goes beyond that, into long term goals, too?

That's another important aspect that Systema helped me to understand, that training is a lifelong journey. It's not that you should train all your life to achieve perfection, not at all. You must train all your life to evolve and adapt. Your Systema must change as you get older, the reason is very simple: if your body and psyche change as years pass, it's logical that your Systema must change too. What you were able to do at 20, your body won't be able to do at

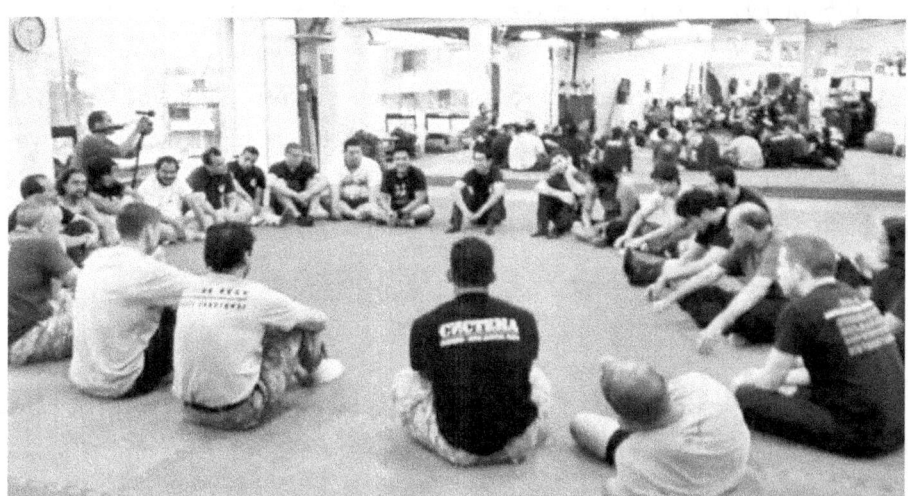

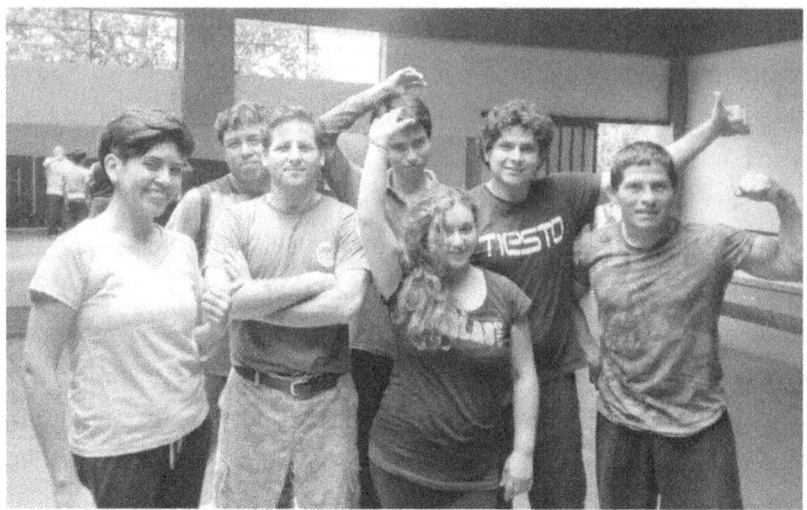

40 or 60. The only way in which your Systema can adapt to the abilities according to your new age and physical condition is by constant training, all your life. You change, your Systema changes with you.

Have you also learned things through teaching?

Yes, teaching Systema has allowed me to learn a lot. Teaching is not just about sharing with others your knowledge and experience (limited in my case) to help them develop their abilities, but, at some point, it's a fundamental and mandatory role one must assume in order to keep learning and evolving.

Teaching forces you to really strive to understand Systema's principles, methodology and goals; and explain them in a clear and enjoyable way. It's not just about mimicking movements and repeating catchy phrases to impress your students. Teaching should be a sincere and selfless endeavor. And yes, sometimes it will be frustrating and challenging, but also gratifying when you and your students progress and grow together. Just remember, you cannot explain Systema with words only, many things should be explained through movement and sensations.

What advice would you give to Systema students?

One piece of advice I give to my students is to "enjoy the process". Most people, when they begin to train in Systema, are too focused on finishing a "technique". They want the end result and this stresses their psyche and, therefore, their movements become jerky and inefficient. They want to "win" as fast as possible and their only gratification is subduing their "opponent". They are eager to know, but not so much on learning. They need to understand that learning is a process, and knowing is the unavoidable end result of that process. Each "step" of the process must be consciously and carefully understood, experienced, and enjoyed. I usually make a comparison with eating. If you just want to finish your plate, just swallow, but you won't enjoy your food. You have to taste every mouthful, feel its flavor and texture..., enjoy the sensations. It takes an appropriate time to do so, it´s a process. If you swallow too fast, you won't taste it; if you chew it for too long, it will become tasteless and dull.

Do you also find that people want to go fast, at first?

Yes, and I advise to them not to train for speed. People are too impressed by speed, they just want to be faster, faster, and even faster. Speed is the consequence of a relaxed, smooth, and comfortable movement. And you don't have to be the fastest, you just need to be fast enough according to the situation. Timing, on the other hand, is a skill one must strive for. Timing is the ability to select the precise moment for doing something for optimum effect. It's a broader concept that encompasses speed (using the appropriate speed, not just being the fastest), and other factors such as distance, direction, depth, and momentum.

Do you have any last thoughts for the reader?

Understand that Systema allows you to develop abilities to defend yourself in an effective and efficient way, but it does not make you invincible. This is why you must take into consideration that a confrontation is the last option. Remember, fighting isn't good nor bad, fighting isn't necessary or unnecessary... but it's always dangerous.

SYSTEMA VOICES

TAHITI

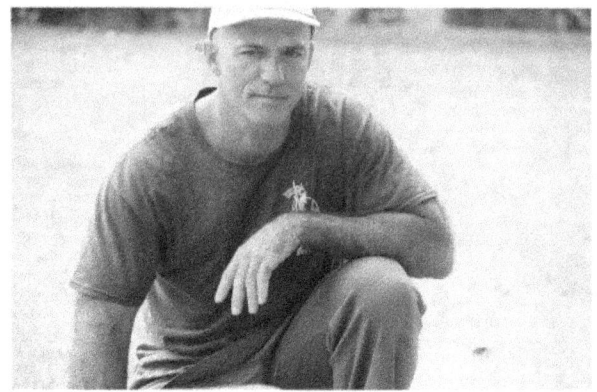

JEROME LAIGRET

Can you first tell us something of your background?

I was born in Tahiti, I practiced Judo as a kid, then I practiced and taught Kung Fu for some years. I also trained in some Krav Maga and other things.

When did you first hear about Systema?

One of my instructors mentioned Russian martial arts to me. I had heard about Sombo but not anything else. However, I figured that as Russia is the largest country on the planet they must have some interesting things! So I travelled to Toronto Camp in 2007 with my backpack and met Vladimir. What surprised me the most was how all the people were so nice, so efficient, no matter their age, size or physique. What I liked also was that the work was not just physical, it was psychological as well, plus anyone could train in it.

Camp can be quite intense, how did you find that as your first experience of Systema?

By the end of the week I admit I was quite lost! I was thinking *what is this System, it is quite surprising!* (laughs). I would hear Vladimir telling me all the time "just breathe, relax, move and stay straight." Then he would show something, I would try, then go back to him and ask more questions. Again he would say "stay straight, relax, breathe,

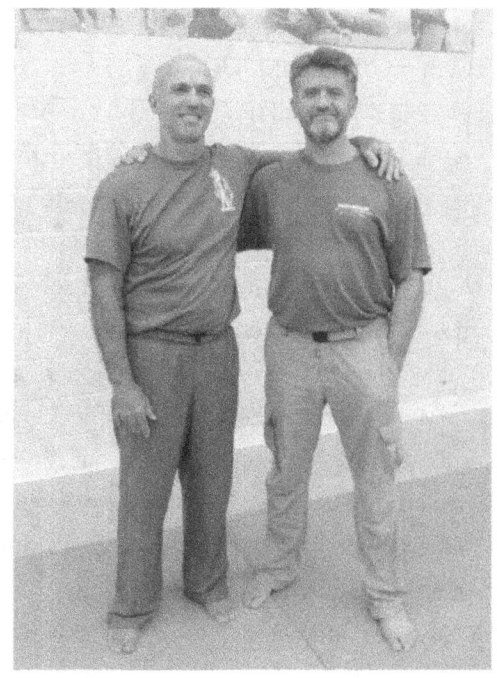

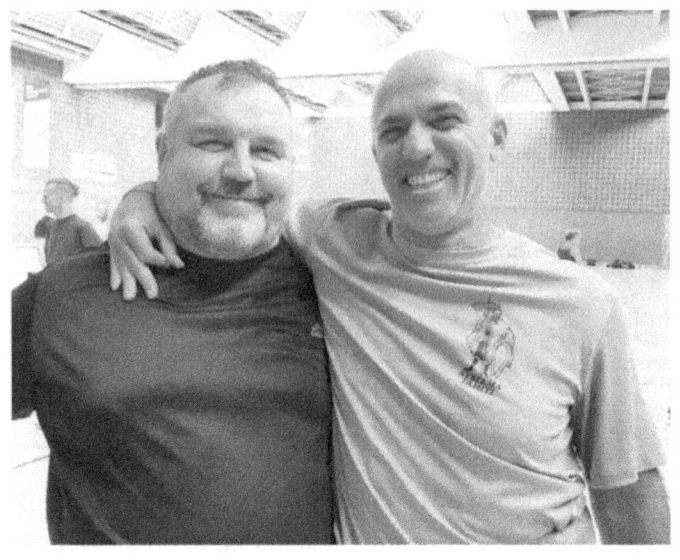

move." He must have told me this a thousand times, then in the end I thought, well maybe I should try and understand what he is telling me! Because I was so used to learning techniques, to memorising kata and forms. So on the way back home I began to study my body, to focus on my breathing, to see how I could move and react more naturally.

And from there you decided to continue the training?

That's right. I went back to train with Vladimir the next time and I remember he told me, "If you really want to progress you should begin teaching." I thought, well, how can I do this, I don't know much about Systema but I shall try. So when I got back home I found a couple of guys who wanted to train. For the first few months I had to pay the rent of the space myself, but I believed so much in Systema and its huge potential that I carried on. Slowly other guys started coming in. In Polynesia we have some big "Maori" guys and they like to see if something is really efficient! So that was interesting, to challenge myself, how am I going to deal with these guys? But it all worked out okay and the school began to grow.

We opened Systema Tahiti officially in 2010 and now we are up to around thirty regular students. That is nice as we can now also run workshops with visiting teachers, such as Sergey Makarenko, Kostya Poshtarenko, the Twins and others. This is good as geographically we are quite isolated. I think we are probably the most remote Systema school! The nearest country to us is New Zealand, which is about 4,000km away. Toronto is 16 hours by plane!

So it's important for us to keep informed, to check out videos. I write to Vladimir for advice, I keep in touch with other schools, I travel to different seminars, it all helps to keep us in the loop.

Does that mean you sometimes have to be more creative in your work, do you think?

Yes, you get creative. And Systema really helps with that. Not only from a martial art perspective but my life in general changed. I found I had a different way of looking at people; my wife, my family, my work colleagues. My attitude changed, now I always say to people, you only have one life, so make the best of it, enjoy it. It's not about fighting, it's about avoiding fights, about surviving and knowing ourselves better.

Do you think this is a major difference between Systema and other arts?

People often ask me "What is better, boxing, Krav Maga or whatever?" I tell them it doesn't matter what is "better", the thing is to find what suits you better. We are all ageing, so as I age I want to move well, to breathe well. Just feel good and ready for any situations ! We should all breathe as much as we can, it is free! (laughs).

Is there a strong martial arts community in Tahiti?

Very strong. They are good fighters and perform well in boxing, Taekwondo, Jiu JItsu and MMA. They like to fight, they are always ready! And as I said before the Polynesian guys are usually quite big.

So how do you deal with that when they come to your class?

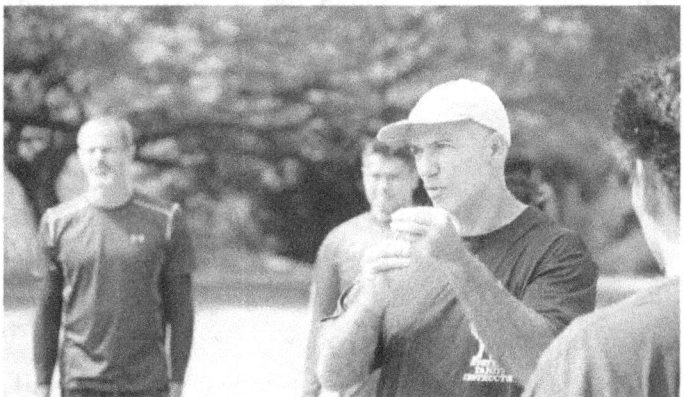

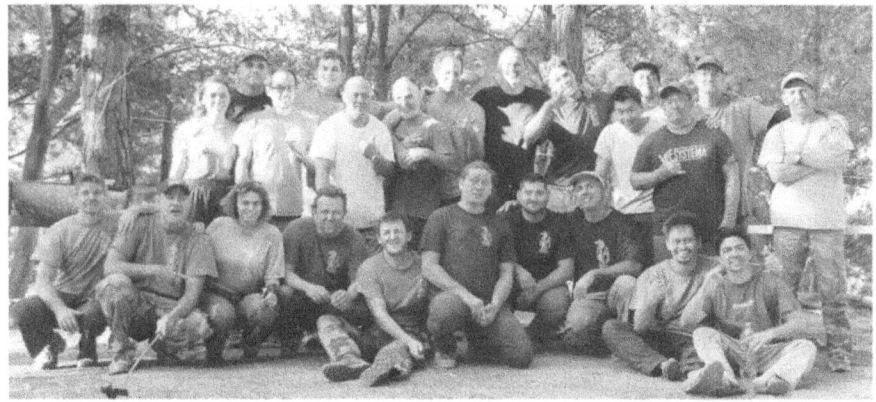

Well if people come and want to try us out, I always start with a breathing session. I find everyone listens to advice about breathing. Then maybe we will work some strikes. It is interesting, these guys often are not keen to be hit. They like to hit people but not to be hit. After that, they like the work or they don't, so they may come back or may not. But it is interesting for me, because you start to learn how to handle such big, strong fighters..

So the approach is less about meeting a challenge head on and more about helping people understand themselves?

Yes. And you know, another thing is people sometimes ask me, "How come we don't have grades, how come we don't have rewards?" I say the best reward is for yourself, not something that I give you. We are what we are, we all do our best with what we have. I think one thing with the island life, is that it is very much more relaxed. People from the cities always seem more stressed out.

The pace of life is slower?

Yes, well it is hot all year round. I mean sometimes it gets very cold, you know 18 degrees (laughs). There are no real seasons, so you don't notice time passing by so much. We train in a gym but also a lot of outdoors training on the beach, under coconut trees, it's gives a different perspective, for relaxation and to feel better our environment, it is ideal. We are very close to nature. Our oldest student is a Chinese guy, 78 years old! He does all the training, all the punching he can still do the splits. I asked him, "How did you come to Systema". He started with us at age 73, he told me, "Well I have an objective. I have a project planned, so I want to be here ten years from now." So that's great, that's the secret to longevity, right? Always have projects, even small ones. Always keep going, once you stop it's over! Keep on moving!

And are your classes all men or do women train with you too?

Women come to train and I found it a bit of a challenge to begin with. Because quite often they do not like to be touched, don't like to be rolled on. Yet I think Systema is ideal for womens' self defence, they are usually more relaxed and move much better than men. But sometimes there is a resistance to contact, they lack confidence in that area. That is something we should talk about more, I think, to get more women involved. Although having said that, when we were showing some massage work with the whip and breathing exercises, the women were usually much more receptive to it than the men.

You find there is a strong reaction when you show work with the whip?

Yes, of course some people instantly think you are a sadomasochist! You have to explain the purpose of the exercise and how it is to help you to really relax. I found it was the women who enjoyed it the most. Their reaction to the pain was very interesting, quite different from the men. Perhaps women have a different understanding of pain than men do?

But once people experience the massage their outlook changes?

Well, when Sergey was over last year, we had a guy come along who is head of a major company in French Polynesia. He's around 40, very athletic, but very stressed out. He asked me to whip him, so for around forty

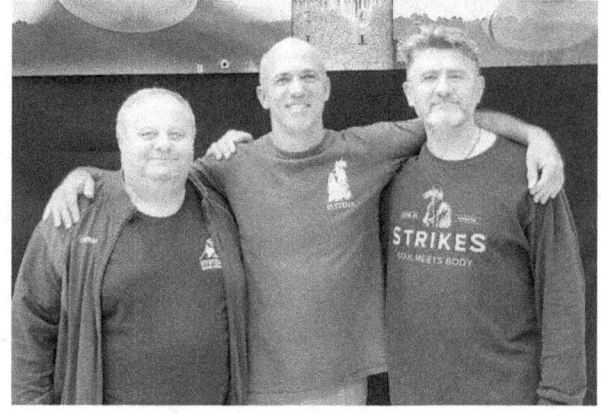

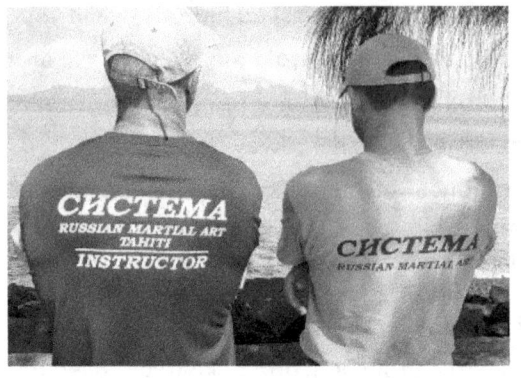

minutes I gave him the whip massage. When we stopped he went away and cried, then came back later and said, "Thank you". It was very interesting to see this powerful guy freeing himself of his stress and tension. It's very satisfying to be able to help people in this way. Even just with breathing and massage you can get very emotional effects.

Do you also teach children?

Well kids are the future for everything, so yes we should get more kids involved also. But the difficulty we have in promoting Systema sometimes is peoples' perception. People can be concerned mostly with how they look. They see some video clips perhaps and say, "But I don't want to look like this person." I have to tell them I'm not asking you to look like this person. You can look however you want to look but achieve that in such a way that you can stay relaxed. Systema can give you a great physique but in a safe way that will not destroy your body. Plus, of course, you have this incredible movement that you can do your whole life.

Do you find a lot of younger guys are more interested in MMA, perhaps?

Yes, so people might ask, "Is Mikhail an MMA champion?" for example. I say no, he's not, but you can always test him out for yourself. When you think about what he can do, you have to ask how many MMA fighters are still active in their 50s?

You mentioned earlier about training outdoors, is that important to you?

One thing on the Islands is that we are very close to nature. We are surrounded by sea, the Pacific Ocean is all around us. And for Polynesians our energy comes from the ground "MANA", that is very important to us. I love gardening, for example, I spend some weekends digging, getting my hands in the soil, gardening, planting, lifting rocks and stones, moving them around. Just feel the ground ! I remember an incident here a few years back. The dock workers went on strike and a Karate guy, a champion, thought he could sort things out. They said to him be careful but the Karate guy was very confident. He went to kick a docker, the guy just picked him up and broke him. These guys are lifting heavy things every day, for them this is a very natural movement!

Is modern technology having much of an impact on the lifestyle?

Well we have Internet and other things, but the Islands are still quite natural, I think. And it is interesting to see how people there, who have never been to a workshop before, react to the training when we bring teachers over. They relate to it very quickly, they like it. Some of our people are very experienced too. For example I have a friend who is a military Krav Maga instructor who has now come over to Systema. He told me he thought Systema was much smarter, you use your brain and your intuition much more. That's the creative aspect again, this is the art, Systema is the art of living.

Have you developed an interest in Russian culture since starting Systema?

I am learning Russian at the moment. I think it's good to be able to talk to people in their native language, it will help me to understand more, I hope. I think Russia has a very interesting culture and their approach to martial arts is fascinating. I got a little tired of people thinking martial arts can only be Asian. Systema proves that is not the case and there are others things too, of course. Bruce Lee was great, but he mixed in many things, fencing, boxing, for example. English people are good fighters, same with Germans and Russians and Arabs. Everyone has been fighting for centuries (laughs).

So what are you plans for the future?

Well I want Systema in Tahiti to continue and to grow. I always tell my people I won't be here forever, I hope others can continue and develop it once I have gone. I hope more kids come in, because as I said, they are the future. To me it is a big family, I hope we can all make Systema grow.

UK

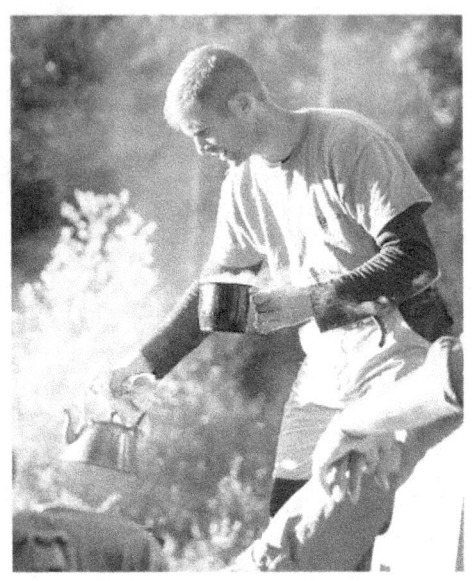

MATT HILL

Let's start with something about your background.

I'm from South Wales, the oldest of five children. I grew up in a small village, with lots of family around. As a parent, I now appreciate how lucky I was back then to have that network of aunts, uncles and grandparents so close. I lived there until I did my A-levels, then moved away at age 19.

When did you start your martial arts training?

I was always interested in physical endeavour. As a kid I was always climbing trees in the woods, pretending to be Robin Hood or King Arthur (laughs). Before "martial arts" broke out these guys were, and still are really, our own British martial artists. I think there was a period when Eastern martial arts came in and were seen as "proper" arts, while our own, historical arts weren't. But history shows that the knights of Europe and the like were very effective.

So as a kid I was always running around with a sword or bow and arrow, play fighting, wrestling. I always loved the physicality of a challenge but equally was also drawn by the mystery and allure of what was beyond that, your character, for example. I didn't realise at the time but that was always important to me, I guess, having a sense of character and depth about you rather than just being a fighter.

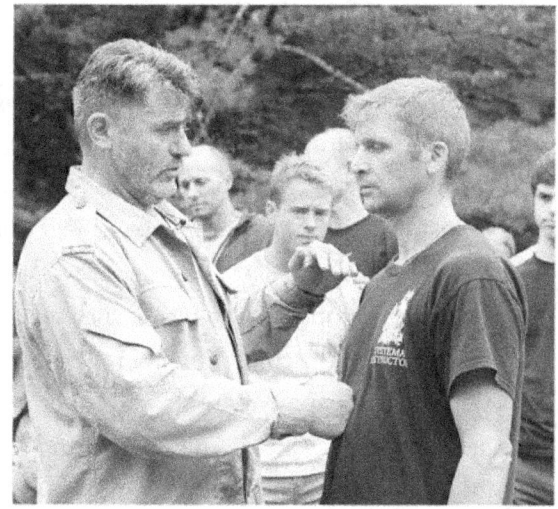

So naturally when David Carradine appeared in Kung

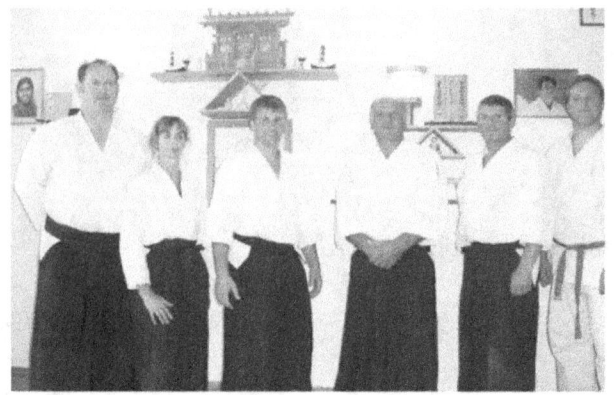

Fu, with his moral code, along with those old British heroes I was fascinated. At around 14 I joined a Karate school, the style was Wado-Ryu, I did that for two years. Then I saw Steven Seagal's first film, Nico, and thought wow, what's this? I'd never seen the multiple attacks before. I discovered it was Aikido, then discovered that there was a guy teaching Aikido in my home town. Mike Narey, he was a 5th Dan at the time, an excellent martial artist and mentor.

I started Aikido at age 16. I took to martial arts well, I'm quite fortunate in that I can watch someone and copy their movement quite quickly. So when it was a martial art with blocks and a shape and a style, I could pick that up pretty quickly. I think that if you get early success in something you are more likely to stick with it, and so I was hooked on martial arts. I was the youngest and quickest person to attain a black belt in that organisation.

Then you moved away from the area?

Yes. I'd done my A levels and was planning to go to University. I took a gap year. A friend and I had a plan; we were going to travel across Canada for three months. That still left some time, so I thought I would throw myself into martial arts and go and study Aikido full-time somewhere. My teacher used to host a teacher from France, Philippe Voarino, he taught a full weapons syllabus as part of his Aikido. When he came over next I had a chat with Philipe and he advised me, if I was really serious, to travel to Japan. He offered to give me the necessary introduction to his teacher but told me it would be more than a three to six month commitment. That meant I wouldn't be able to go to University. I spoke to my parents and other people and got differing advice. But the best advice was that I didn't have to make a quick decision, I had a few months in Canada to think about it. So we went ahead with the trip and the plan was... to cycle all the way across Canada.

Cycle! Not motorbikes?

No, pushbikes! (laughs). All the way across and back again. In three months! My friend Brendon and I went over there in March with these massive boxes containing our bikes and had the first couple of nights in a hotel. Money was tight and a friend had an Uncle living in Toronto, he offered to help us out and put us up. I remember sitting round the table at his house, there was this map on the wall behind him. He asked us about our plans, we explained what we wanted to do. As we were talking I kept glancing up at this map, slowly realising it wasn't a map of the world, it was a map of Canada! He asked if we'd really thought our plan through (laughs) and so we ended up changing it. We stayed with him and his family for a few days, lovely people, and we left the bikes in his garage. Instead, we hitchhiked. It was a good decision! We bought a big union jack and stood with that on the side of the road. Some of the drivers were ex-pats, a lot of them had family back home, and we met some really nice people. I think we ended up only using the tent for one or two nights, the rest of the time people put us up in their homes. People there are used to driving long distances and the roads are not that busy. We could wait hours for a lift sometimes, so when someone gave you a lift you could be with them for most of the day! We'd get to know them quite well and they'd invite us home to meet the family, it was great.

One guy and his wife were school teachers. They were doing Shakespeare at their school and asked us to go in and read for the kids, with the genuine accent! We stayed the whole day doing a tour of all the classes! The whole journey, we didn't have one bad

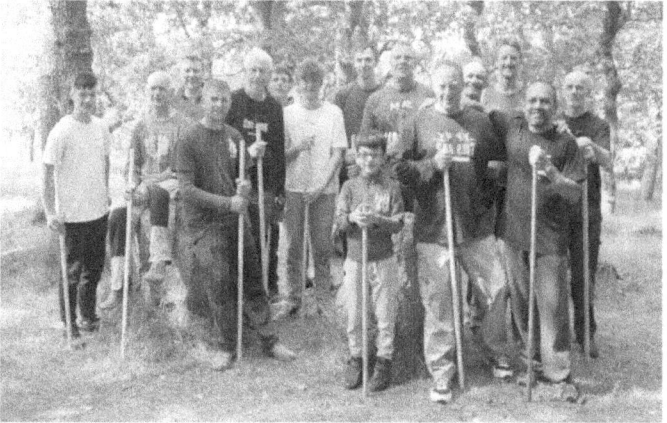

experience, it was an amazing trip.

And at the end of that had you made a decision about university?

Pretty much everyone I spoke to in Canada said the Aikido offer was an opportunity that might not come round again, so I should take it. I made the decision to go to Japan. I returned to the UK in June and in November flew out to Japan on a one way ticket, that's all I could afford. I had my letter of introduction, directions from the airport and enough money for one month! I'd heard it was quite easy to get work teaching English out there.

When I arrived, I found that wasn't the case, so after the first month I had to make another decision as I was running out of money. My parents came to the rescue. They had been putting aside some money per month for me into a savings fund and this fund matured whilst I was out there. It was just enough either for a flight home or to stay for another month. I decided to gamble and stay another month. It paid off, I got some extra work teaching English and ended up staying in Japan for two and a bit years.

How did you adapt to Japanese culture? Did you find it very different?

Yes, hugely. I got on well but had to change myself a lot. It helped that I'd made a good first impression, which is very important over there. I'd learnt how to greet in Japanese, took the teacher a gift and followed the etiquette. At the time I think that to get on well there you had to take on the customs, the mannerisms. I learnt to speak Japanese, I became a live in student, which meant doing all the work, the cleaning and so on. I was the first Westerner in more than a decade to be taken as assistant to Sensei on an overseas trip, that was a huge honour and privilege, a big thing, it was quite an emotional experience.

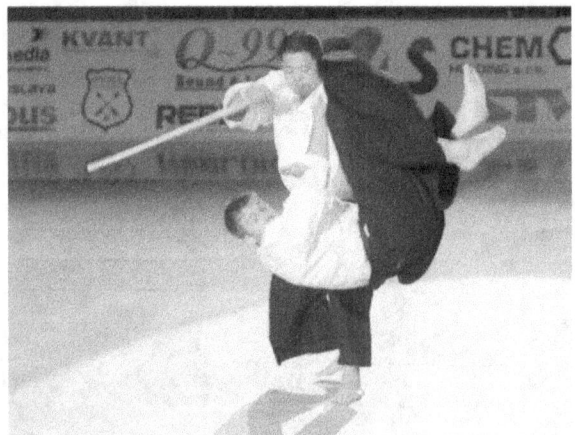

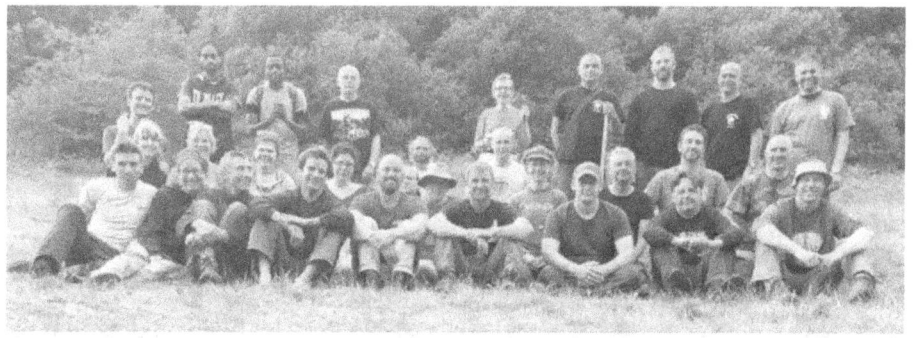

When you returned to the UK, did you find you needed to adjust again?

Yes, that was a hard re-adjustment! Trying to fit back in was difficult. Sensei had asked me to open a club and start teaching, so there was an expectation. But I was 22, had no business skills, no real personal skills. I was good at Aikido but lacked the skills to build a group. My only experience was in teaching in Japan, which doesn't work the same in the UK – no smiling, no jokes, no talking! If people were not what I considered respectful enough, I didn't take it personally but took it as an insult to the art. So I struggled. I was hugely confident in my Aikido ability but my personal confidence was rock bottom. Looking back, in Japan I'd been a big fish in a small pond in a very different culture, not just Japan, but *old* Japan. Here I felt like a fish out of water culturally.

So I tried for a couple of years, then went back out to Japan. I thought I'd give it six months and decide if I wanted to live there permanently or come back the UK. I'm not one to make quick decisions and five months and two weeks in I still hadn't made up my mind! Then, with two weeks to go an Australian guy turned up at the dojo. It was my job to welcome new people and when chatting to him, I noticed he had a British accent. He told me he'd spent eight years in the UK, in Aldershot. For some reason I just said "Oh, the home of the Paras!"

Did you have family who had served in the military?

No, not at all, no military background whatsoever. I'd watched a documentary on the Paras in the 80s, but that was it. A couple of nights later I was chatting to him again after training, he told me he'd spent five years in the Paras and three years in SAS. As soon as he said it I thought, "Yep, that's

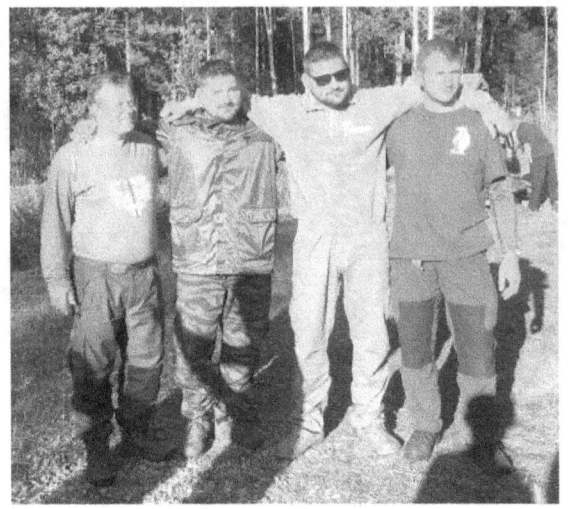

what I'm going to do." It was the oddest feeling, because I'm not a knee-jerk reaction person at all, but this was very intuitive. I'd never even considered it before, the military had never been on the radar but in that instant I made up my mind. He advised me to try to go via the Officer entry route, as I already had the basic qualification requirements. Then over that final two weeks he kind of downloaded all the advice I needed to give me the best chance of getting through the interviews and selections.

I imagine that's a tough process?

Well I got through the careers office interview first, and then you do a two-day intensive selection with the Regiment/Corps that you would like to join. For me that was The Parachute Regiment. That was the hardest physical thing I'd ever done up to that point. If you pass that you then go onto a two day officer selection with the Regular Commissions Board in Wiltshire, and if you pass that it is followed by another three day selection. So there are all these points where you can fail.

They look at your complete character, your intelligence, your cultural breadth, your ability to lead, to handle problems under pressure, your determination, you get tested on all these things to see if you have a chance of passing the rigours of training. Anyway, within nine months of getting back to the UK I was starting at Sandhurst.

Was the Army what you expected? Did it give you what you were looking for?

Well the decision was really a gut instinct one, so I wouldn't say there was anything in particular I was looking for. But when I stand back objectively, I guess I'd always been interested in developing myself as a person, as we were talking about earlier. I mean, I knew had weaknesses in me, and Sandhurst was a great place to have those weaknesses pointed out by people who could first find and then help you deal with those weak points.

From a martial arts perspective, I'd done the old school hand-to-hand stuff with Aikido; and this was a chance to understand martial arts in a modern context, to live a warrior life as a professional. It answered many questions, but I was still looking for something when I came out and that was when I found Systema.

So when did you first find out about Systema?

I first heard of it in my last year in the Army when I was a Company 2IC in Lichfield. I used to get e-mails from a guy called Stanley Pranin, now sadly passed. He wrote an article called, 'An Encounter with Systema' about the first time he went to Toronto to train with Vladimir. He wrote about how he'd never seen any of the drills and exercises before and that the level of natural, spontaneous skills was very high. He didn't talk about techniques at all; and this sounded very different to the Aikido approach. He said it was based on principles and an adaptable skill set and this adhered to my military experience. He was intrigued by this and said that Vladimir was not only highly skilled but a kind and generous person too.

He also wrote about the background, the military and how it was often practiced outdoors. That kind of tied a lot of things together for me, it resonated so much with what I'd already done. At the end of the article was a list of seminar dates and Mikhail had a seminar coming up in the UK very soon. I enrolled

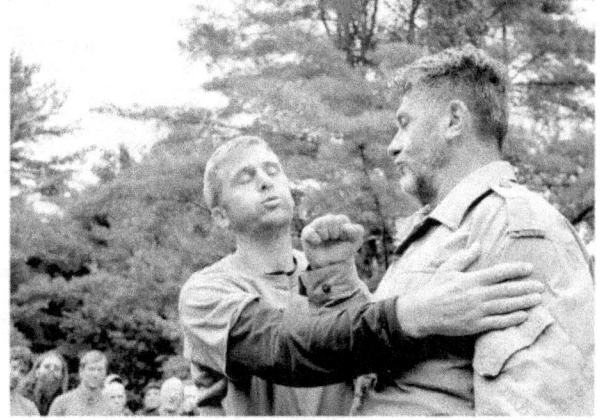

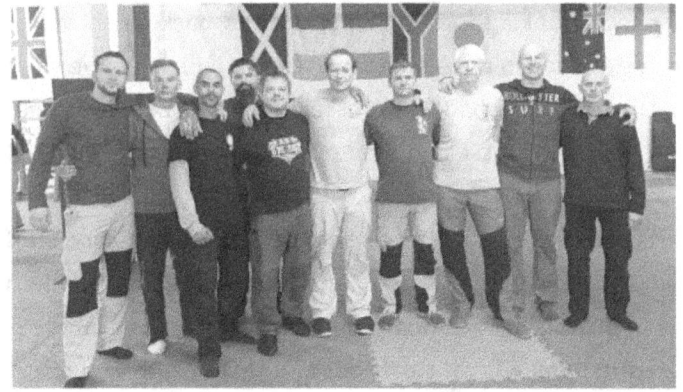

on that seminar. Vladimir was there also along with some of the UK guys. I remember thinking that it was so nice to go in anonymously, no one knew who you were, I loved that, I just immersed myself. I was able to observe and study it.

What were your intial impressions on seeing it first-hand?

We did all the usual exercises, you know, walking and breathing, squats, press ups. I was thinking okay, it's a bit weird but it's okay. Then Mikhail came over and asked me to attack him. When I look back this was another of those two or three profound moments we have in life. I asked how to attack him, as I was used to doing in Aikido, he said, "doesn't matter." So then I asked how fast, he said, "doesn't matter."

I came in with a punch and he didn't knock me into next week but just kind of gently tipped me up. I remember lying on my back looking at the ceiling thinking, "what happened?" It was interesting, people had thrown me thousands of times but I'd never felt anything like that. I remember having a huge smile on my face as it brought to mind something that my teacher Morihiro Saito Sensei had told me. Morihiro Saito had been a live in student of Morihei Ueshiba (the founder of Aikido) for 23 years and was very close to him. He had told me when he first met O'Sensei, the founder of Aikido, he had the same experience. His explanation was exactly the same as what I had just felt. It was like a meeting of different worlds across different times. In that instant, any doubts about Systema were cleared from my head. Then I heard him talking in the Q&A at the end, which I liked too. Another thing that struck me was the accessibility and openness, so I was hooked.

Were you teaching Aikido at that time?

I was still in the army at that time, and hadn't taught any Aikido, apart from two sessions: one baton and restraint session to the guys in 2 PARA before we went to Northern Ireland and another on a pre-Sandhurst course, when someone asked me to do an interest session.

So the idea that military guys learn all this amazing hand-to-hand stuff doesn't really hold up?

Not in my experience, because anyone who's trained in martial arts knows how long it takes to build proficiency and the Army doesn't have that luxury of time. Nearly all your time, even in elite forces, is spent perfecting your ability to work as a team and with weapon systems. You work as part of a buddy pair, fire team, section, platoon and company etc. There is no point in spending much time teaching people to work without weapons. You don't even spend much time using your handgun, at least in most parts of the military.

How does that sit with the modern background of Systema?

That's the interesting thing. Roll forward four or five years, I had Mikhail and Vladimir over for the *Legends of Systema* workshop. I was driving them to the seminar from London and I asked the question, because I was curious. I had no doubts about Systema and its methodology but I couldn't see how that had developed through the military, as I have said they just don't spend much time on hand to hand, in fact they work to avoid it. Mikhail answered that it depends which part of the military and began to explain about SMERSH and counter-intelligence teams. As soon as he explained,

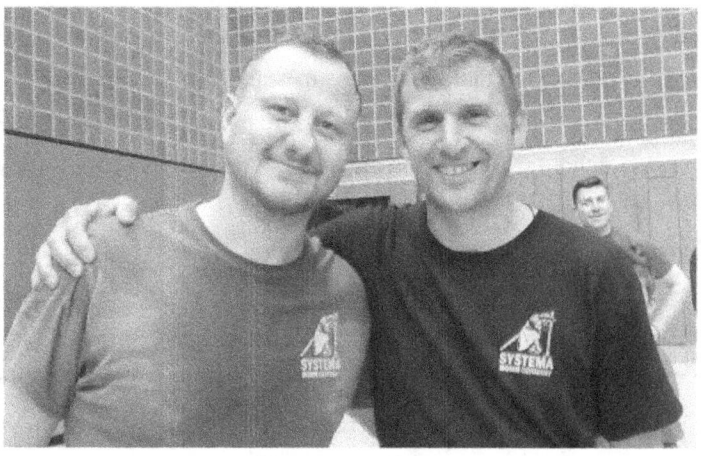

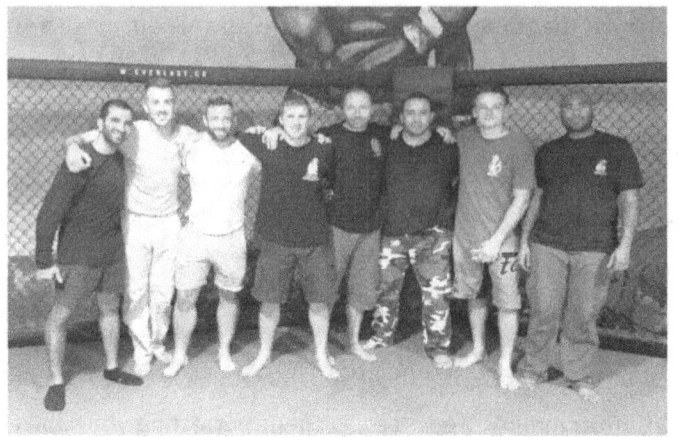

then everything clicked, especially about staying calm and the breath work. Because generally you don't train soldiers to stay calm – I mean you train them to stay calm enough to operate and listen to commands, but in the main it is aggression that will get men out of cover and storming a position.

But when Mikhail explained about the need of counter intelligence services to operate in public spaces, in plain clothes, to notice things, to investigate, not be detected, to move through a crowd, to follow people, and also to operate hand to hand, then it all made sense.

No one who has lived through war would ever dream of glamorising it. Yet it remains a huge part of our culture and entertainment. Why do you think that is?

I think that the idea of heroes is so deeply ingrained in our DNA, in our ability to have survived as a species or as individuals. I mean it's only the last couple of hundred years you've not had to worry too much about safety when walking down the street. We are descended from survivors and that desire to explore, to fight, to have adventures, to develop skills and to admire those who have them is in-built. The story of the hero stays strong, even now when there is so much contest about 'just' wars and war being politics by other means. But it's still the guys on the ground who get up and do the heroic things, I think it's in-built in us as men and women to admire that.

There is a kind of glamour to it, look at the movies, they are archetypal stories, facing evil, rising to the challenge, it's in every myth and culture. Through that process of slaying the literal dragon they find the literal gold, which in the analogy isn't actually really gold of course, the same as the dragon isn't really a dragon. The dragon is that deep fear that we have to find the courage to meet and the gold is the transformation of ourselves in this heroic endeavour, becoming stronger in character, incorruptible, like gold.

Was leaving the Army similar to returning from Japan?

In many ways, yes. Because in the Army you are very well looked after. You are kind of in a bubble. Rent is taken out at source, you are fed, there's a great community, camaraderie and so on. However, I didn't find it an issue when I left the Army, perhaps because I'd already been through that coming back from Japan.

Another aspect of people leaving the armed forces is PTSD and the like. Do you think that Systema can be useful in these case? Or just in life in general?

Firstly I would imagine it is rare to find anyone in this life who doesn't have some form of post-traumatic stress. It's a spectrum; everyone gets triggered by certain things from childhood or what happens to them as adults. Being bullied is a traumatic experience for anyone, for example, so most people can relate to that. With soldiers it can be more extreme, of course. What has really surprised me is just how effective the tools we have in Systema are in managing that stress. Both when it's coming in and when it's triggered. I remember reading (I think either from Mikhail or Vladimir) about warriors having to do difficult things in the course of their work and the monks teaching them deal with that, how to cleanse themselves, so that they are able to work effectively the next time.

I was interested in why I'd never come across that in the Army, in any Army. There are some inbuilt mechanisms,

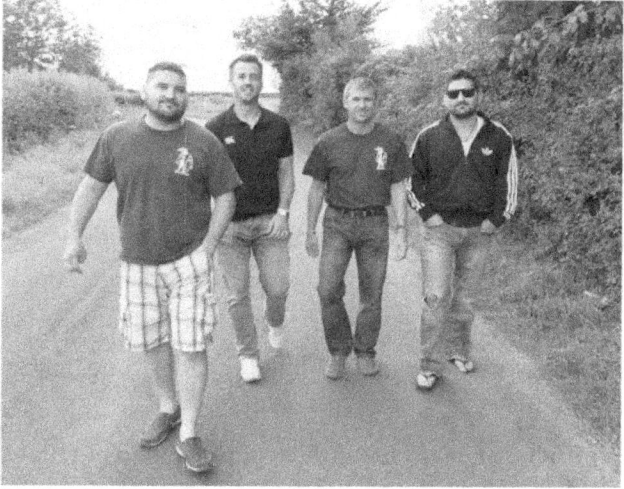

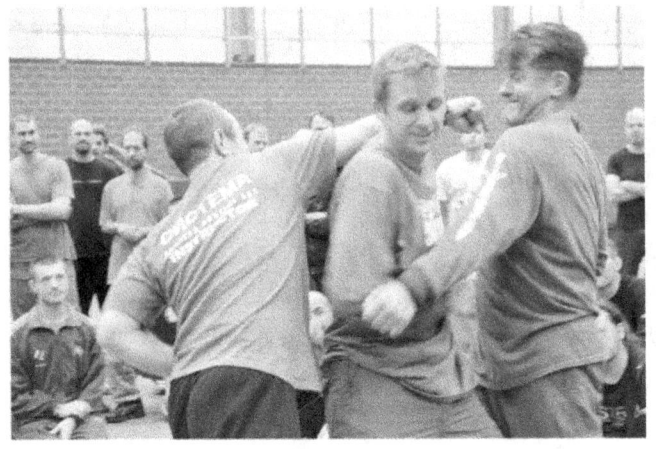

such as the strong camaraderie, the drinking culture. There's pre-tour leave and post-tour leave etc. But I think that it is changing now, it used to be very male-dominated, there was a framework in which men were able to be men, with their own ways to deal with things. But society is changing, we are much more open, able to air and talk about things, the role of men in the world has changed; in my generation even, you see it everywhere, in the workplace, in family relationships. Whether it is for better or worse we don't know yet. We haven't run the experiment for long enough.

Systema really has incredibly practical tools to help with PTSD. I've seen it in classes; I've seen it in myself. I'm working with a Clinical Psychologist at the moment, putting together a program for stress management to take into companies. The problem is most people associate relaxation with some kind of outside agency or vice, a drink, maybe drugs. They have no idea how to bring that about naturally. For me, the biggest gift from Mikhail and Vladimir is how to transform the landscape in a single breath. The internal and the external, because how you are also affects the people around you.

Do you think that Systema can have a role to play in bringing people together?

Yes, because the thing we are deeply understanding more and more now is that nothing is in isolation. Every good or bad thing you do has an impact somewhere and that impact can resonate out. I think that the more people we can have walking this Earth calmly and influencing interactions in that way, the better. I read Vladimir say that for a long time he wanted to teach people how to fight, now, if he can teach people to truly relax, that's enough. That's profound on many levels. For someone who has that amount of skill to say that, it's something else.

How do you get that across to people though, especially in today's social media dominated world?

It's hard, because no one trusts a panacea! However, because Systema is an operating system, it seems to make you better at whatever you do, even if it's just walking down the street. I mean we have to market ourselves to some extent and I think Vladimir and Valerie do that really well. They have helped me a lot with that too. They give a lot of advice to new Instructors, they deeply care. The difficulty is that exercise now tends to be more about what you look like rather than how healthy you are. In twenty years I've no doubt people will look back and wonder why people went into a windowless, forced air environment to run on a machine. People think of health and fitness as the same thing but that's not always the case. Take running, people suffer in their running, and most hate every minute of it. Perhaps there's a better way. It's something I wrote about in Living Systema. Why do you want to get fit? What do you want to achieve?

You mentioned earlier your interest in outdoor training, how have you brought that in to your Systema?

When I left the Army I had a job that involved travelling. I was in South Africa a lot and met Vadim Dobrin over there; I went to his classes and had private sessions with him for about eight months. He talked to me about running outdoor camps. He's another ex-Para so we got on well, he's a great guy, I learnt a lot from him. After that, I went to Vladimir's camp in 2012

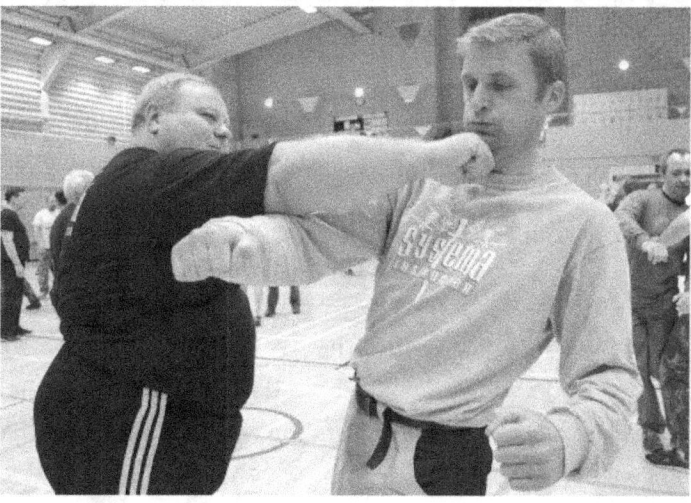

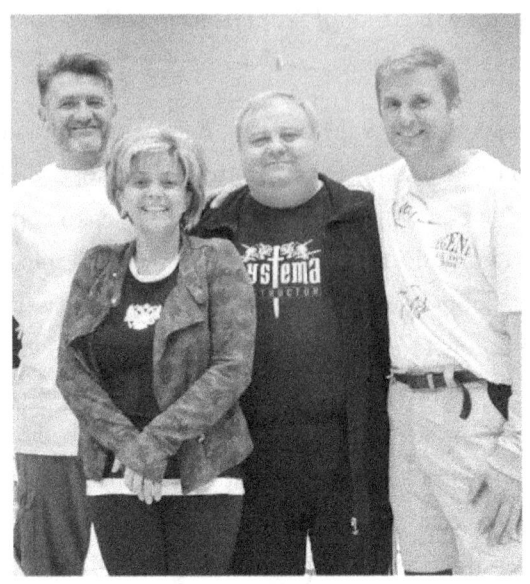

and it just struck me: *why have I never trained outside in all this time?* For me, this stuff was born and grew in an outdoor environment, why take it inside and train in a sterile environment? It comes to life outside. I noticed in my own camps, people get things quicker and they go so much deeper so much faster. Even sitting down and getting the fire going is a lesson. So everything about it made sense, from a health perspective, a functional perspective, an immersion perspective.

Also the stripping away, the disengaging from the cyber-hive. People can get emotional at the end of camp, people understand on some level that they've gone back to their roots, perhaps. I think the further we get from nature, the further we get away from what it is to be human. In a lot of ways we've done to ourselves what people have done to animals by putting them in captivity. We've put ourselves in our own zoo, look at all the mental health problems around these days. We've lost touch with the reality of things. We rarely get cold; we rarely have to do things that are distasteful like killing and butchering our food, though someone, somewhere has to do it. We are diminishing ourselves with comfort. It's interesting to speculate where that is leading.

We live in interesting times?

Absolutely, for example I heard that the Orthodox Church in Russia has had ten million new followers in the last few years. Here, we've had a swing away from religion but I think there's a danger of throwing the baby out with the bathwater. Our laws, our culture the way that we deal with the big things in life has all been based on our religion. There is a tendency to think that we are "cleverer" than that now, but there is an understanding of human nature that we need, because life is hard. It doesn't matter who you are, you can't be permanently

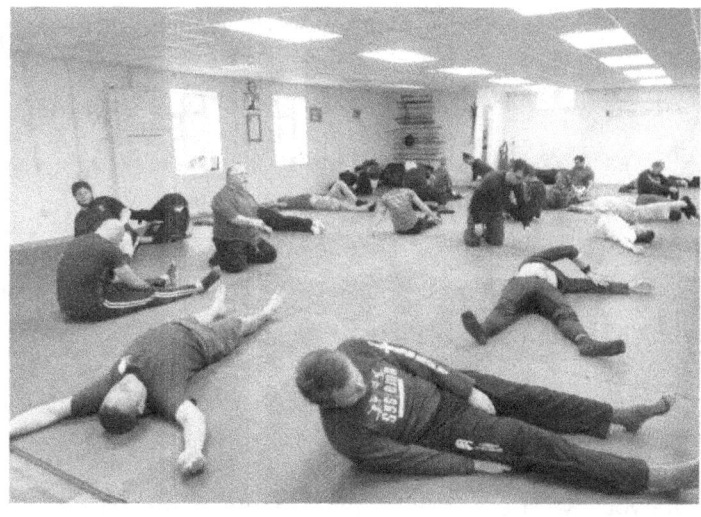

happy. Unless you know how to pick up that burden and walk with it you'll have a hard time.

When did you start teaching and how did you find it, at first?

From the time that I came out of the Army and saw Systema, my Aikido began to change. I guess at the start, before having had contact with Vladimir, I thought of Systema as sloppy Aikido with some strikes in it. I loved the creativity of it, so as soon as I started teaching again in 2005 I added in the breathing, the Four Pillars and the strikes, things that I'd not seen in Aikido. After the camp in 2012 I came back and made the decision to split the two. So half the class was Aikido and half was Systema. I didn't want to mix the two anymore. Then I began to realise that I couldn't ride two horses. I also had an opportunity to go full time, so I called a club meeting and told them I would just be teaching Systema. They were nearly all Aikido people, but almost all of them stayed with me during the change. It renewed my passion for teaching, because in Systema I find you get people coming in very quickly and saying what a difference the training has made in their everyday lives. One lady explained how she had to walk up seven floors at work every day and she always had to stop to catch her breath. Then, once day, she did Systema breathing and didn't have to stop. It's a small thing, but it's a big thing, too. Teaching helped me improve my own skills of course, but seeing the effect on others was a real boost. I started with two nights, now I have nine classes a week at the Academy.

You have a full time school now?

Yes I have a full time Academy in Melksham, Wiltshire. I teach daytime and evening classes for children, ladies and adults. I split the classes between Health (the Systema holistic approach to breathing, movement, fitness and relaxation) and Martial Arts. It is only me in there, so I can be very flexible with class times, running workshops, and one-to-one training.

Given that Systema is wide in application, where do you start as an Instructor?

In the beginning I think it is it's hard to work off the cuff. Because you are nervous, worried about material, about running out of drills. So having a bit of structure in the beginning is helpful. Now, after teaching circa 20 hours a week for 6 years as a full time instructor, and for many years previous as a part time instructor, I may have a plan but it always changes. You know the saying: '*no plan survives contact with the enemy.*' So, to use a military analogy, there is a plan there in the first place, and having a plan allows you to adapt. My lesson plans are similar, I have an idea of what I am going to teach, but that always changes depending on who is in the class and their needs. I think that the more experience you get the more flexible you can be in helping someone to understand what they need to make the next jump.

Because it is about teaching people to understand rather than to just copy?

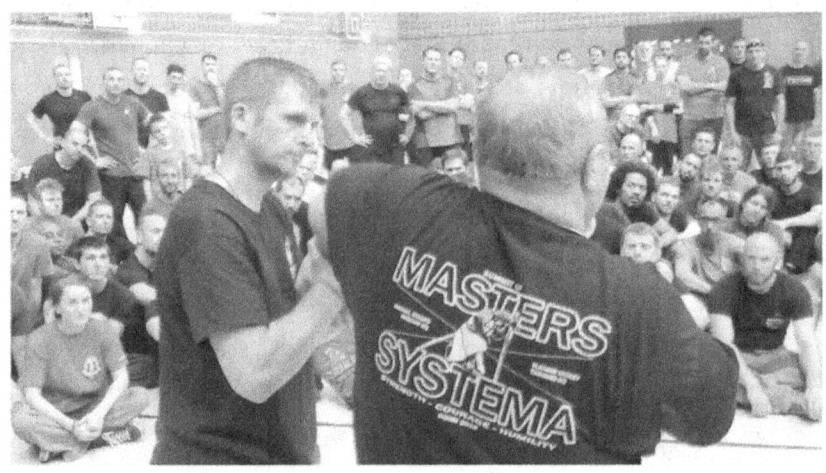

Yes. For example this month we've been doing some of the strike work and I've been showing the guys that it is a feeling. That feeling is not attached to a particular form. Once you have that feeling you can attach it to any shape, so you have

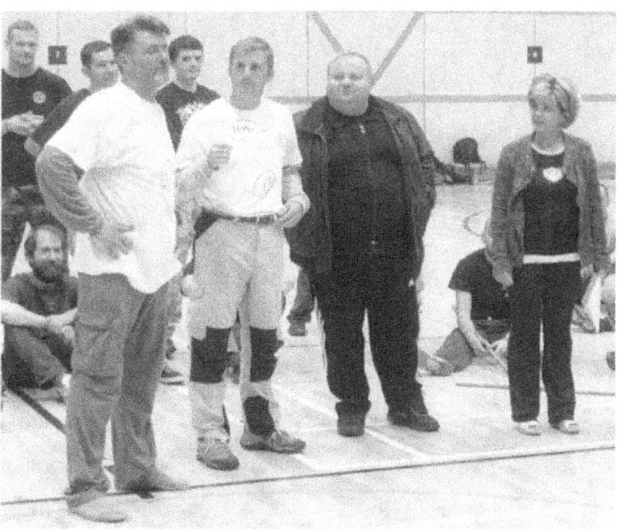

an infinite number of options. If you go form first, you have an answer to maybe a couple of problems and people can get lost or hung up on the form.

You mentioned books earlier, when did you start writing?

Writing a book was a suggestion from a friend who was filming for me. We had some stills at the end so he suggested using them for a book. It wasn't something I'd ever contemplated, so I asked people in the club what sort of things they'd like to see. As I'd split the class between health and combat, I got two sets of answers so it made sense to bring out two books: *Systema Health*, and *Systema Combat*. One covers breathing, movement and health, the other is combat drills. I approached them along the lines of being the sort of thing I'd like to have when I first started training. I brought those out, then later, after thinking about how your Systema only really improves if you integrate it into your everyday life, I decided to bring a out another book on that subject. That was *Living Systema*, and we put out some on-line videos to accompany these books as well. It's nice to see that books as a medium are still valued, too.

Compared to your previous experiences in Japanese martial arts, how much do you think that Systema relates to Russian culture?

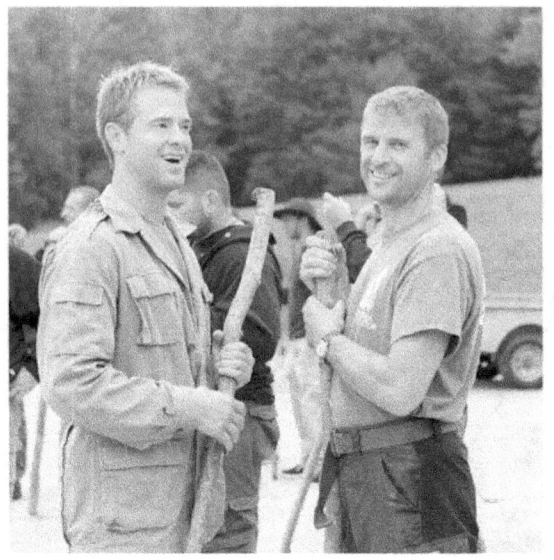

That's an interesting question. Definitely, with Japanese arts many people are drawn to the culture and the aesthetic. But I'm not aware of anyone who has come to Systema because they wanted to learn about Russian culture, it certainly wasn't something that occurred to me, I was attracted by the skill and character of Mikhail and Vladimir. Perhaps the military angle attracted some at the start but I don't think those people lasted for long.

One thing that I do find is that Eastern European people seem to get it very quickly, they get how something like breathing and relaxation can sit right next to combat work, they understand that. Maybe part of that is because, certainly the people I've met from Russia, and Eastern Europe, tend to be very family orientated and rooted in community. That also ties in with an outdoor lifestyle. People think of outdoor folk as tough, hard people, and they are. But a true outdoor lifestyle has a lot of sensitivity involved. You can live the illusion that you can crash through any situation but put someone in the jungle or forest and try crashing though. You wouldn't last a day. The softness with which even the Army moves through that environment is telling.

You have to have a balance of hard and soft. In survival there is a real sensitivity and softness of spirit that you need to prevail. You have to be able to read things, to stop, listen, feel things. That blend of hard and soft skills is the only thing that works in reality.

You mentioned the Orthdox Church earlier, is that something you have been drawn to?

Yes, but it took me a while. I'd seen how Vladimir dealt with situations, the compassion and the humanity. Likewise, when I met Mikhail. That was something to aspire to, I thought. The seed was first sown when I hosted them in the UK. I asked Mikhail what I needed to do next to improve my Systema. I thought he would give some advice on breathing or movement or how to improve my strikes, instead he said I should read the New Testament! After my initial surprise I did and it called to me in many ways. It always had in truth. I have always been drawn to spiritual and philosophical things. I sat on that for a couple of years, then on my third trip to Toronto I asked to be baptised. It was an amazing experience; Vladimir is my Godfather, as he is for many people.

Now, I try to go to church as often as I can, it's the most peaceful, calm and relaxed I feel. I'm still very young in it but for me, really, the whole of my Systema journey has been like coming home. I think that if you were born in the UK and raised in a village community you were probably raised in the Church of England ethos and lifestyle. You know, weddings and funerals, prayers and hymns in school assembly, but apart from a few dalliances never in any more depth that that for me.

Then with martial arts I was drawn to Shinto, Buddhism and meditation, that was a big part of my life in Japan. So it all just came together really. It was a feeling of coming home, in a martial and spiritual sense. When I was making the decision to just teach Systema, it was a big decision. I had a following in Aikido; there was loyalty to my teacher, twenty-five years training, the finances and so on. It took me a long time to reach the decision, but in the end it became easy. I realised Systema was what I had been looking for all along; it was one of those realisations. Then those two things fit so perfectly together; what I had been raised in as a child alongside the martial aspects. It made sense to me. That's where I feel at home.

Any final advice for the reader?

If you can find a local school, go along and look at the teacher but also look at the students. You should feel comfortable in a good class. For learning, relax, soak it up and start to notice in everyday life how you breathe, how you move and how you approach situations. It's not how well your doing in class, but how differently you live your life.

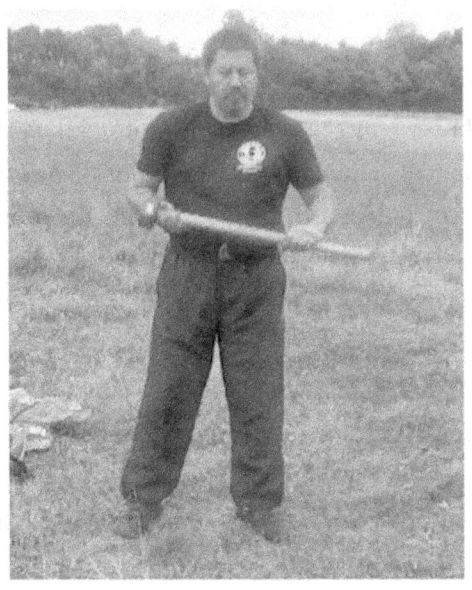

ROBERT POYTON

Can you first tell us where you are from and something about your background?

I was born and raised in East London. My parents were normal, hard working people, with a big interest in sports and music. I lived in London until I was in my 30s. It was an interesting time and place to grow up.

In what way?

Well, there were a lot of things happening in London in the 70s and 80s. A lot of street politics, marches, protests and the like. There was a very vibrant youth culture, especially during the whole punk era. And things could often turn "lively", especially at football matches, or even most places you went on a Saturday night. Bank Holiday riots, lots of gangs, street crime, all that type of stuff was going on.

Do you have any military experience or military background?

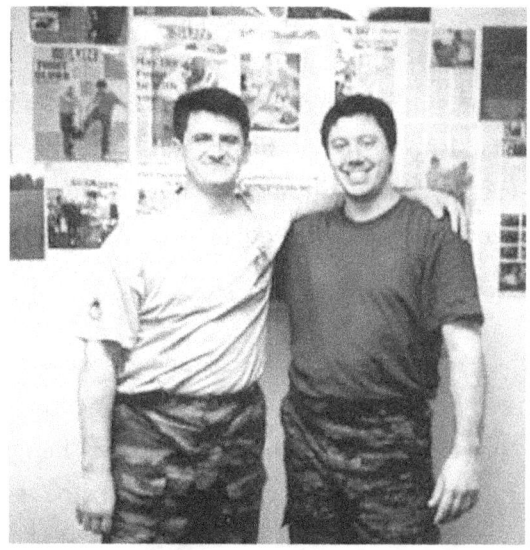

No, though, of course, various older family members served in and experienced the war. In fact, even growing up twenty years later, some parts of the East End were still bomb sites from the Blitz. My Dad did his national service in the 50s and I always had an interest in military history but the armed services were not a family tradition. Having said that,

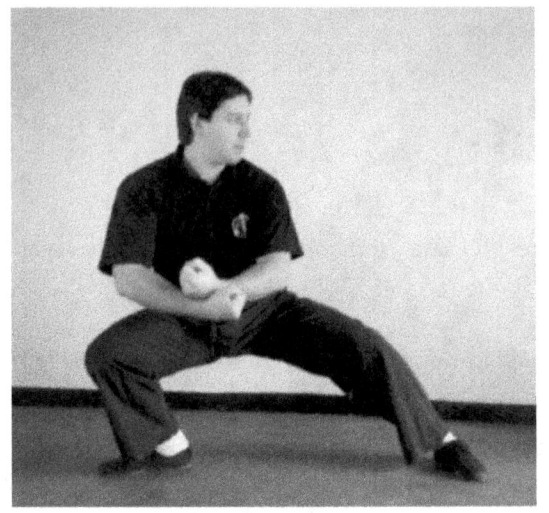

most of the men on my mother's side were coppers, they were quite a big police family, I guess. The family on my father's side... well, let's just say that they were definitely not police! (laughs)

What was your first exposure to martial arts?

My dad took me to Judo classes when I was about seven. I also did some boxing, that's kind of a tradition in East London, I suppose. Then what really sparked my interest, as a kid, was seeing the Kung Fu TV series with David Carradine, followed by the whole Bruce Lee boom, of course.

So you started training in Kung Fu?

Well no, because at that time it was difficult to find a class! I remember going to the library to get more information and back then, they had one book on Judo and one book on Karate! I'd already done Judo and Karate didn't appeal to me. It wasn't until a couple of years later that I saw a local class advertised for Tai Chi Chuan. I didn't know anything about it, other than it was "kung-fu", so off I went. The teacher, John Ding, had a background in Shaolin and Preying Mantis Kung-fu and had begun training in Tai Chi a couple of years before. Luckily, it was a traditional Yang family school rather than one of the more exercise-based off-shoots.

It was very traditional type training, then?

Yes, it was old school. Stances, form, conditioning, that type of thing, that was one aspect. But what also grabbed my interest, from that TV series, was that there was this whole philosophy behind it too, this "ancient wisdom." I think that had an attraction for many people back then, when these arts still had a lot of mystique attached to them. Having said that, we were very much rooted in applying the stuff. A group of us used to get together on a Monday night at an old gym in the grounds of a local hospital and try and work things out, how could we use this move against a punch, what if someone did this, that kind of thing. It was all quite crude, we had hardly anything in

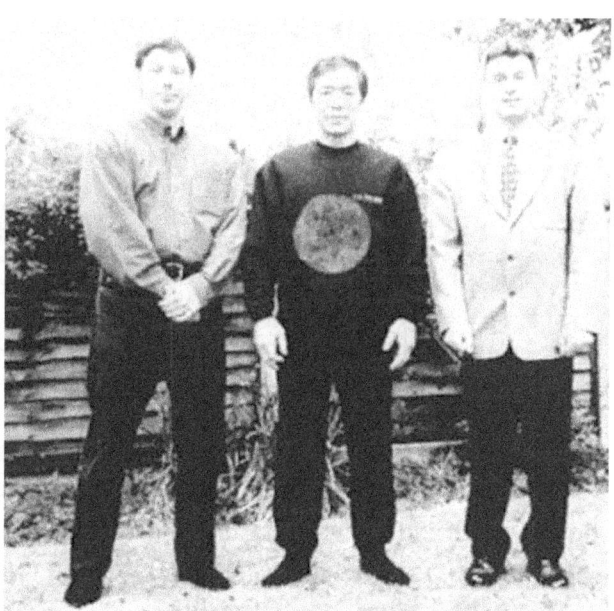

the way of equipment. Maybe some sports gear, like cricket pads, I remember using phone books as focus pads (laughs). But we worked hard and enjoyed knocking each other about.

Did you find yourself having to use what you'd learned at all?

Now and then. Like I said, back then wherever you went it was easy to find trouble. By that time I'd left school and had become a full time musician, mostly playing the London circuit. To earn some extra cash I started doing a bit of door work here and there. Nothing major, as most of the doors back then were run by heavy firms. Mostly I was just helping out friends who were running their own gigs or club nights at different places.

That was good experience, because it taught you how to deal with people verbally. I found on the door you almost had to take on a particular role. A big guy who had the look, for example, could purely be a visual deterrent. Another guy might be the "firm but fair" one and so on. How you presented yourself was important, you soon learnt that you can never show fear. Also, you had to be aware not just of what was going on but also who was who. Handle the wrong person the wrong way and you could be in for repercussions, so it was a fine balancing act at times.

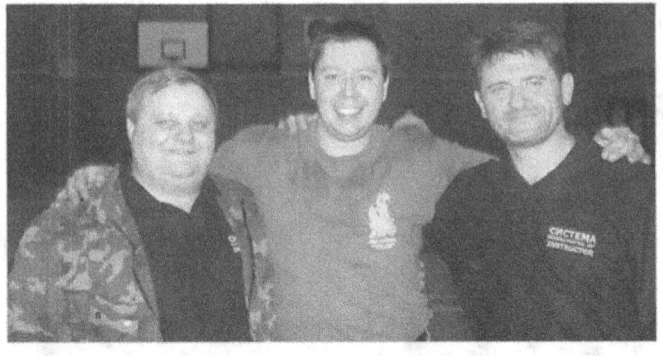

Where you still training Tai Chi then?

Mostly, though I began trying other things too. I had a good pal, Robert Murray, he'd started training in Tai Chi but also did a lot of other styles. His main background was in Wado-Ryu Karate and Ju-jitsu. Rob had a cellar kitted out as a training room in his house in Hackney, we used to get together a couple of times a week and train in different things. We did a lot of bag and pad work, I remember, plus trying out knife defence, board breaking, grappling, anything and everything. There was more information starting to come out by that time, more books, more workshops, things were opening up.

Meanwhile at the Tai Chi school, a group of us were growing more disillusioned, as the tone and style of training at the school had begun to change. Things came to a head and eventually a number of us split off to begin our own school. That was when I began cross-training a lot more.

What sort of things were you doing?

As well as the training with Rob and others, for a few years I spent almost every weekend going to some workshop or another. Things ranging from hard-core combatives with people like Dave Turton, Peter Conserdine, Steve Morris, through to traditional teachers, like Ji Jian Cheng, Chen Xiaowang, through to more fringe subjects, pressure point teachers, people who claimed they could work "no touch" and so on (they couldn't!). Alongside that, I was also practicing various types of qigong and meditation. For Tai Chi, I trained for a while with Jim Uglow in London, then began getting Vincent Chu over from Boston. He was my last Tai Chi teacher and the best one in many ways.

Where did you first see Systema?

Well I started putting all this stuff together to try and make a "complete" style. By then I was also working with Dave Nicholson, we'd met when both judging at a competition and started exchanging ideas. Dave had a school up in Yorkshire, so we merged our schools together and set up our own association. We used to go back and forth to each other's clubs, as well as teaching workshops. We were always looking round for things to add to our syllabus, to fill the gaps as it were. This was the time when videos were getting more popular, you were now able to see so many more teachers and styles. A friend used to send me tapes and one of them was Vladimir, this was the old TRS tapes in the late 90s, I guess. We were intrigued by his movement and how he worked. It looked to us like all the things the Chinese internal arts promised, but there in one accessible method. However, I thought his guys fell over way too easy!

Anyway, I was interested enough to send off for some more videos. The clips I saw of mass attack work intrigued me. That was the first time I'd seen martial arts multiples work that actually looked like a fight as I knew them from the terraces at Upton Park (laughs). Chaos, no one lining up to take turns, no fancy techniques, just a good old fashioned punch up! That really caught my attention. So we began adding all that into our syllabus too. At the time I was also travelling around teaching workshops at various schools, Karate and Kung Fu clubs mainly, so I had a great opportunity to begin testing this new material out - in a friendly way, for the most part.

And when did you first get to train with Vladimir?

I think it was a year or so later, I saw that Vladimir was on his first visit to the UK, so Dave and I went along. Vladimir was very friendly and his remarkable ability was obvious. The first time

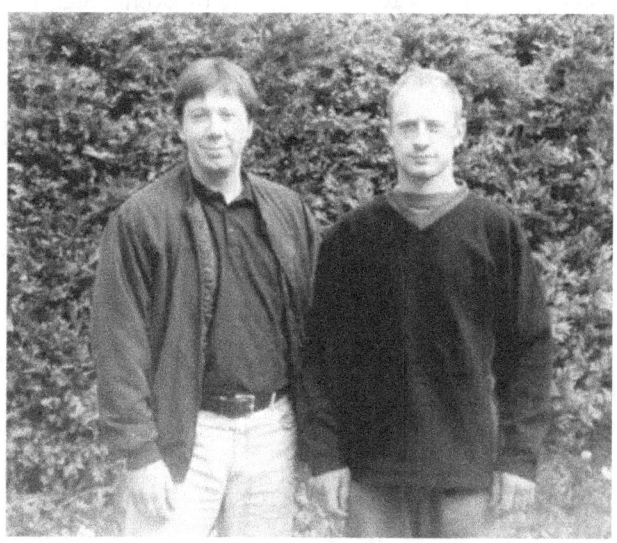

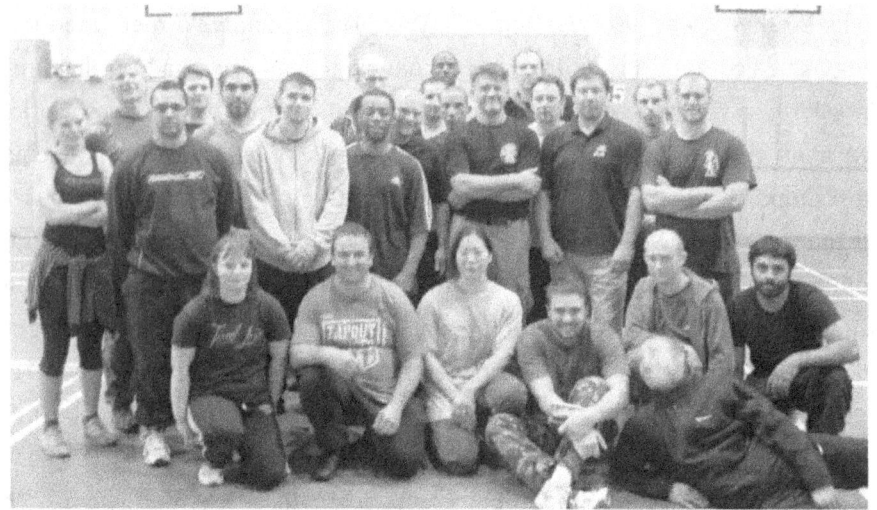

I got "hands on," he asked me to try whatever I liked, so I went in to clinch. With my Tai Chi push hands background, that was my strong point – I thought! Three times he put me on the ground, it was effortless on his part. The third time, he said, "Your balance is very good!". Well, I had to laugh. I'd never felt that before, you understand? I mean I'd met lots of people better than me, but when they worked with you it was always a struggle. They might pull off a good technique, but you could feel it happening. With Vladimir, there was just a sense of falling and I quickly revised my opinion about his students going over too easy! But that aside, there was not a hint of dominance or showing off. Sometimes, teaching in different styles, you found people who felt they had to prove something or who'd try a cheap shot to establish their dominance over you, you know how it works. But Vladimir was so gentlemanly with it, not only that but, of course, he then started showing us how he did it. So that was it!

Did you then begin Systema training?

We still tried adding things in to our own syllabus for a while but for me it got to the stage where I thought I'm adding so much in, why don't I just do Systema? To do that I obviously needed a lot more training, so I went over to Toronto.

How was that experience?

Humbling! I felt like a complete beginner again, totally out of my depth, to be honest. But everyone was so patient and generous. Vladimir and Valerie too, they filled a suitcase with video and t-shirts for me! So back in the UK I decided to switch the school over completely to Systema. Of course not everyone liked the change, but I felt it was the direction I had to go in.

You then began organising workshops in the UK?

Well, I'd already been organising workshops for Kung Fu teachers from China and the USA. But yes, my thinking was that not everyone could get over to Toronto, so I invited Vladimir over. The first one I organised was in Cambridge, must have been 2002 I think, and Vladimir brought Mikhail with him! So that was great, I got to work with Mikhail for the first time too, which was an even stranger experience than working with Vladimir.

How was that?

Mikhail asked me to punch him in the face, so I did. I couldn't work out why I kept missing him though. His movement was so subtle, I couldn't see it. Very confusing. Then he hit me back (laughs). I still remember that hit, it made me do the best twisting fall and roll I've ever done. So after that weekend we used to get Vladimir and Mikhail over regularly, as well as Sergei Ozhreliev and Valentin Vasiliev, both also great teachers.

And you were still going across to train in Toronto?

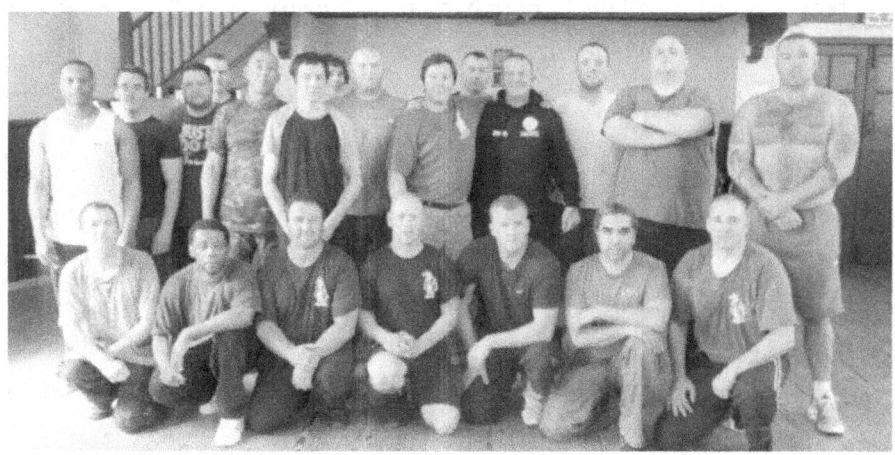

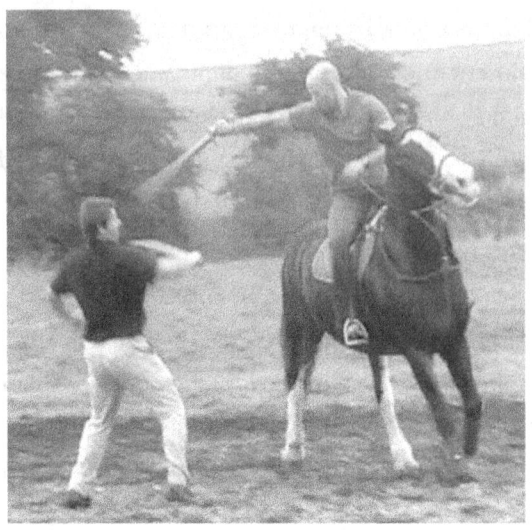

Yes, plus I took a couple of groups over to Moscow too. Those Moscow trips were very interesting, alongside the training we got to see some sights and also experience something of Russian culture and hospitality. For me, those visits helped put the art in context and I began to appreciate that there was a lot more to Systema than I had originally thought.

What was it that led you to training just Systema and not other things?

I'd still occasionally look around at other things, because you can get knowledge from almost anywhere. But I became increasingly aware that, rather than have to study a bit of this and bit of that, Systema was a complete methodology in itself. Because, at its core, it's a study of how you, as an individual work. I often come back to this idea of body systems – nervous system, blood circulation, skeletal, cardio, emotional , etc. We are made up of all these systems and the training teaches you how they work, how they interact, how to harness them. That's one part. Then you learn how your systems interact with others, both human and environmental. Given that, you then have a universal blueprint for dealing with any situation

But you have to train for those situations?

Oh yes, it's not just a matter of doing some breathing exercises then thinking you can fight a tiger! But what you do have is a firm base, a strong starting point. You then train to work those core attributes in the context of whatever type of situation you want. So we've had people working in a swimming pool, for example, or with horses, or outdoors, or in several types of scenario. You can vary the intensity every time as people progress. Each situation has its own challenges but each has core similarities too. With this approach it means that I don't have to study Art A to learn knife, then Art B to learn grappling and so on, I can do it all using the Systema toolbox.

Now when we add in to that the considerable operational experience of the main teachers, plus all the health and other aspects of training, you have something that is as complete and coherent as I've ever seen.

So cross-training for you goes beyond just mixing styles?

Absolutely. And I find that this "completeness" is something that many people are still searching for. The advice you always hear for learning self defence is, "Train boxing, Muay Thai, BJJ." All well and good in some respects, but that's three arts you have to learn. Plus, how do you combine them, how do they flow together? Plus, what do they teach you in terms of awareness, communication, situational work? It's common to see people suggest someone try all these different things to develop skills but they are only thinking in terms of style or technique. This is a very limited approach. It's funny, quite often I see on martial art forums something like, "If only there was an art that combined awareness with striking and fear control and..." Hello! Here's Systema!

Is Systema becoming more popular in that sense?

As far as the UK goes, yes and no. Most young people now gravitate to MMA or BJJ for martial arts, or go into historical sword fighting and that kind of thing. Mainstream self defence is still quite niche, people think of it in terms of a six week self defence course, you know, learn a few techniques. However, I have seen a big growth of interest

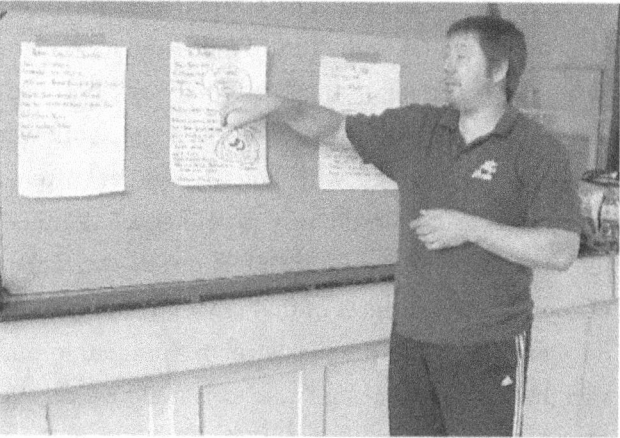

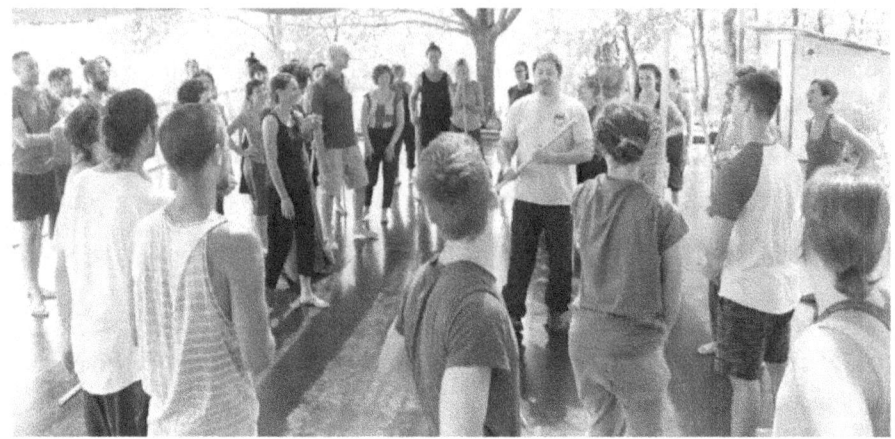

from what you might call the professional sector. We have a considerable amount of people training with us from law enforcement and military backgrounds. For example, just recently I was teaching sessions on knife awareness to Youth Workers and Police Officers up in Leicester. Also a lot of people who come in are experienced in other martial arts and are looking for a new approach. A lot of us seem to go through the same process with traditional Eastern styles!

I've also noticed a recent trend of people adding System exercises into their own styles. Mostly uncredited and, quite often, performed in the wrong way. This is not being honest to your students and, potentially, putting them at risk. There is a problem with some modern forms of exercise or movement, in that the work is presented as a series of "challenges". It's all competitive and macho, it's about image and ego; again, this is a recipe for injury.

I do think that in the future more and more people will either be training Systema or working in the "Systema way", because it is so effective. People don't always appreciate that much of this work was developed by top level professionals, backed with huge resources, often under extremely testing conditions, usually in times of great need. We tend to forget the amount of research and experience that has gone into this work, theory and practice. And, of course, some aspects of that work go back generations. It also continues to develop. It's live! In the mainstream, you quite often find that it is not what is said that is important, but who says it. So we practice things in a certain way and some people ignore it. But when their favourite teacher or sports scientist promotes the same thing, then suddenly it's great!

You have also been teaching dancers recently?

Well this is another growing area, people who are interested in movement in general. I was approached by Bruno Caverna a couple of years back, he's the founder of Formless Arts and Play Fight. He invited me over to Berlin to teach alongside him at one of his workshops and it was a great experience. The students were mostly professional dancers but also some martial artists. Bruno is all about exploring and pushing the boundaries of free movement and what it means to be free, physically and emotionally. He's a very good instructor and it was very interesting for me to view my Systema work through another lens. Since then I've taught around Europe for some different groups and also at Bruno's annual retreat in Tuscany, which is a remarkable ten day event.

How much do you have to alter or soften your teaching when working with dancers?

Not as much as people would think. After all, movement is movement, breathing is breathing, so many of the drills are exactly the same. Some of the emphasis may be a little different, or specific topics may change, but if people think that professional dancers are somehow "soft" they should try one of their training sessions! Believe me, a lot of their movement is quite remarkable and extremely fluid. Plus it was also very interesting to see how many people at the recent event lined up to take punches and strikes with the whip.

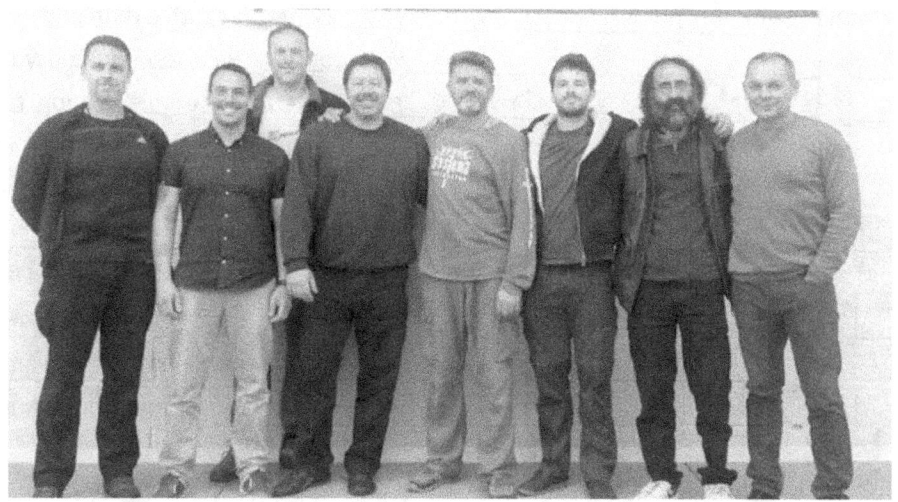

They want to try something tough?

No, quite the opposite. They are perceptive people and see the taking strikes work for what it is – not about being tough, but about releasing tension. You see, people who use their bodies professionally have to learn to be as free of tension as possible. Tension results in injuries, for one, which means that you can't work. So that is one level. If we go deeper than that, people who are creative and who learn to express themselves in different ways, often become quite self aware. This means that as their work deepens they become more aware of emotional tensions and underlying issues. These have the same impact as physical tensions, they are inhibitors to work and expression.

So these people fully understand the need to uncover the issues that others, perhaps, prefer to keep buried. The striking work, when done properly, is a very quick and effective way to do that. Someone once told me it was better than six months of therapy (laughs). Seriously, you can see a change straight away with many people, one guy at the Tuscany camp told me, "You changed my life with a punch!" Although my ability in that field is nowhere near Mikhail or Vladimir, it's very rewarding work.

It's quite remarkable that you can go from teaching security staff and LEOs to teaching dancers with the same method.

Isn't it! But that's the beauty and power of Systema. There may be some who want to classify it as a "martial art. " That's okay, but it's a term that doesn't resonate with me, personally. For me that term has more negative than positive

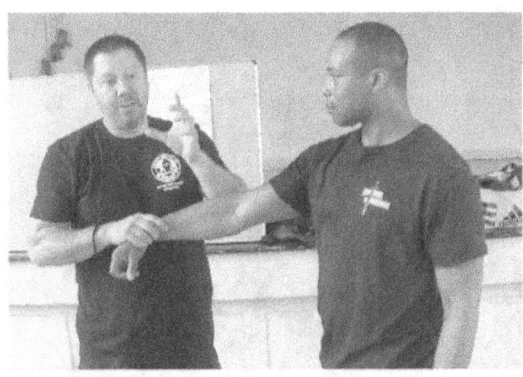

connotations. Why would you want to take this wonderful thing and burden it with a syllabus and grades and a hierarchy and all the rest? Well, each to their own. For me, Systema is much more about personal exploration and being a full functioning and capable human being, fit for any task.

I gather you are now also a published author?

Yes, I have a few books out now. Well, I've always been a writer. I wrote for several martial arts magazines since the 80s, and published my own Tai Chi magazine in the 90s. I have also been making instructional videos since the mid-90s, though they are now downloads of course. Then a while back I thought, why not try writing a book? I did, and some nice people bought it, so I've written some more! Not just Systema books, I've also got into writing fiction, which is great fun and a very steep learning curve. About twelve years ago I also got back into my music, and now have various recording and band projects on the go. Systema helps considerably with creativity, I find.

And you are still teaching?

Yes, but in some ways things have gone full circle. I've been through running a "big school", teaching several classes a week and so on. Also I now find that most of my "old regulars" are busy running their own clubs and classes. So I'm in the process of going back to having a small group of people training with me at the house, working together, trying out some different things. In a way it's a return to those old Monday night sessions, but with better equipment and, hopefully, a bit more knowledge! On top of that, I teach workshops, plus we run our annual Outdoor Camp. I've been doing those in one form or other for around twenty years now and love training outdoors, especially in the forest.

What, to you, are the defining principles of Systema?

To me they are like the four legs of chair, you have to have each of them present and they all have to be the same length if you don't want to wobble! So it's quite straightforward, breathing, mobility, structure and relaxation. I say straightforward but to achieve mastery of each alone is one thing, let alone combined in a fluid situation. This is beautiful work because it is constantly evolving, both to the needs of our situation and to our own needs as we age. These days I prize breathing and mobility above all, that's what keeps you active and young at heart. Mentally agile as well as physically.

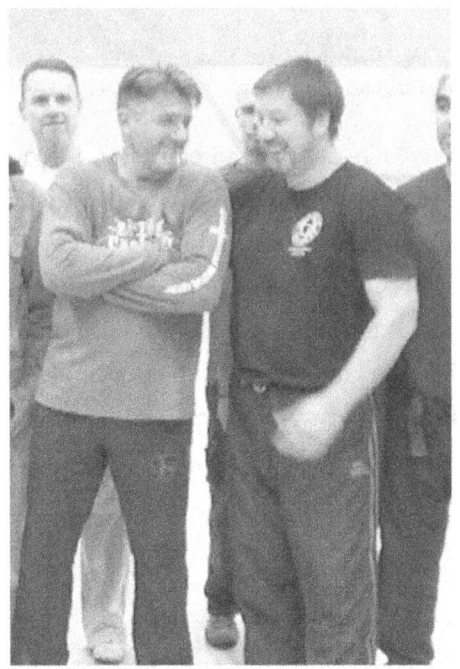

Do you have any advice to instructors on how to instruct their sessions?

At first, it's not a bad idea to have a lesson plan. Later on, you can work much more on the fly. Understand the needs of the group and work to them, not to your own wants and preferences. Be careful to show enough but not to show off, most of all be aware that you are there to teach and to help people. Of course, a teacher also needs to be a student to, so getting regular guidance yourself is very important. It's easy to get stuck in bad habits or dead ends, we all need a helping hand (or fist!) at times. We are lucky these days in that Mikhail and Vladimir continue to teach around the world, plus, of course, there's all the senior Instructors that are available to train with and learn from.

Where is the line between testing and ego?

Our group has always been keen on testing our work. When you say "testing," most people think of padded gear and "all out sparring." Well that is one approach but there are other methods too. You have to find ways to put people under psychological pressure, then see if their skills are up to the situation. So first you have to give people the coping mechanism to deal with the test, don't just throw people in cold. Then you have to find a way to graduate the pressure, in whatever form it takes. And, of course, you have to carefully monitor to ensure we are not going from "testing" into "torture!"

So we have tried a wide range of things over the years, some may seem a bit extreme but if carried out properly they are all useful. Really, padded up sparring may have a use at one stage, but is quite limited and is by no means the be all and end all of testing. As for ego well, we all have one otherwise we couldn't function. We come back to the professional mindset again, keeping

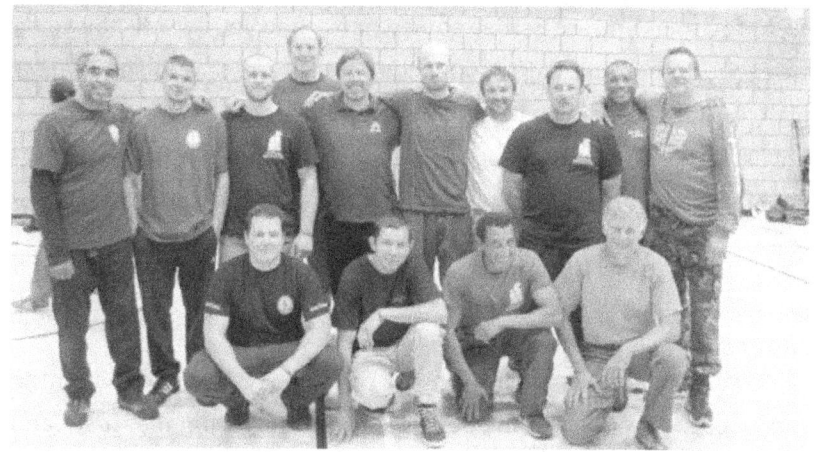

things in the context of preparing people for a situation, not proving to them how great you are. It's easy to put in cheap shots in Systema training, it's easy to try and "win" all the time. Doing both misses the point entirely and pollutes the training. I've always told people that the purpose of the drill is not to defeat the purpose of the drill! Given the way we train, without mats and so on, injuries or other problems have been very rare. I put that down to the Systema mindset - we are there to help build each other rather than just ourselves. You also learn just how fragile you really are!

How important are the cultural aspects of Systema? Or is it more universal?

In comparison to my time in the Chinese styles, not very for me. I fully appreciate the historical and cultural background of where Systema comes from. I'd also say some aspects of that culture, the Orthodox Church in particular, have had a profound impact on my life. However, in practice and application, I feel Systema is universal. It's the most human system I've seen in that respect. No jargon, no animal imagery or shamanistic overtones, it is purely human. I was previously extensively involved in various meditation and occult type practices and, for me, they led to a dark place. Systema brought me out of that, onto a much more positive path. But of course, each of us has to find their own way.

As your training goes on in Systema, do you appreciate the depth of it?

Absolutely, the more I train the less I feel I know. I'm just scratching the surface. You think you are getting somewhere, then you see Mikhail doing some amazing work that just baffles you! It's very interesting to see the potential though, to have examples here and now of where the art can lead. So many martial arts rely on stories of legendary teachers from centuries past. We have living, breathing masters who are here and now and willing to teach.

Any stories you would like to share about your experiences with Vladimir or Mikhail?

I'm sure everyone who trains with either has plenty of interesting experiences to recount. But my personal favourite is from that first Cambridge workshop. Dave and I went to Heathrow Airport to collect Vladimir. The arrival of the Toronto flight was announced and we were positioned just behind the barrier, directly in front of the doors through which the new arrivals came in. So passengers began coming through the entrance, no Vladimir! We were thinking, oh no, did he miss the flight, when Dave says, "He's behind us!". Somehow, Vladimir had come down the passageway, through the doors and to around behind us without us seeing him, he was laughing! I later asked him about that and he talked about how people have gaps in their awareness, gaps that you can move into. That's a fascinating area of work to me, awareness, perception, how we see things and how that can be influenced.

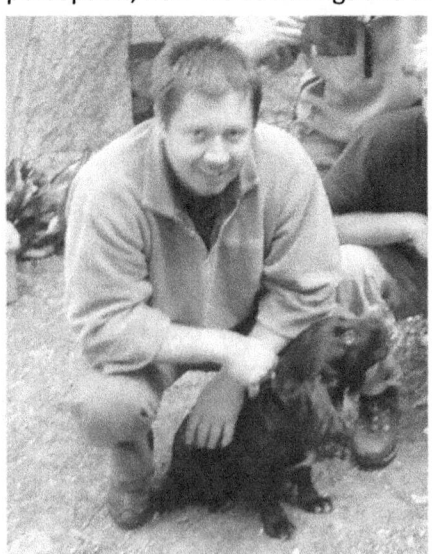

A bit like a magician use distraction techniques?

Well that can be part of it and for a while I studied mentalism, magic tricks and similar things. Occasionally I like to drop one of those tricks into a session, just to show people how easily they can be fooled. Of course, I always show how it is done. I think this is important, teaching people to spot when they are being manipulated, and to be more aware of what is going on around them. Again, the outdoor training is great for that.

Camouflage and concealment?

That's one aspect. But on a more general level, just being in a live environment, with uneven ground, obstacles, poor weather and so on. It takes us back to a more natural state, I think. There's something I read a while back too, which resonated with me. It was about when they first started training Commando units up in Scotland in 1940. A trainer from the time wrote that the best candidates they had were either Scottish ghillies (gamekeepers) or Cockneys (people from London's East End). Both were very used to living off their wits, acting stealthily, thinking outside the box. You see, people often think of camouflage and hunting only in a rural environment but all the same principles apply to an urban environment, too. Blending in, keeping sharp, being able to adapt and so on. Again, I find that a very interesting area of training.

Lastly is there anything you would like to add for the reader? Any advice or thoughts?

The two most important things in training are intelligence and consistency. Understand why you are training, what you are doing, ask questions and, when appropriate, analyse. Of course sometimes you just need to let your body work, but you can analyse later. And be consistent in your training! If you go to class once every six weeks, don't expect to advance very much. At the very least, if you can't make class, do something every day. Some exercises, some breathing and movement, test yourself in some way. Make Systema part of your everyday life, not something you just do at training. That way you begin to live the art, that's when it really begins to work!

USA

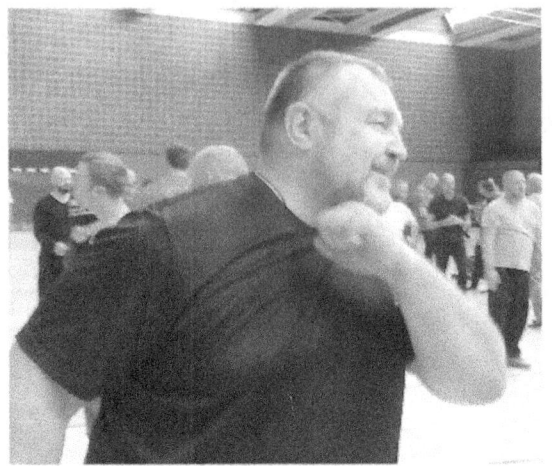

SERGEY MAKARENKO

Can you first tell us where you are from and something about your background?

I grew up in Moscow, a town called Lyubertsy, known as the criminal capital! I was never involved, though, and actually I had a good childhood, I first got into sports at school, around 8th grade. I started freestyle wrestling at first, at school, then Karate came in but it was soon made illegal. So it was a double pleasure, to do something forbidden!

So you had to train in secret?

It was very secret training, yes. It was something very different for us, we were used to seeing Sombo, Judo, wrestling and so on. Boxing was the only striking sport that we knew, so Karate became very popular, though it was underground. It was fun, we were breaking boards, breaking bricks, hurting each other a lot! There was no semi-contact then, it was all full contact, no one worried about that. There were a lot of injuries (laughs).

Were you still training in wrestling, too?

I started doing Judo and Sombo at college, then when I came to the States I discovered that the rules of the Judo schools there were very different! You could not do arm

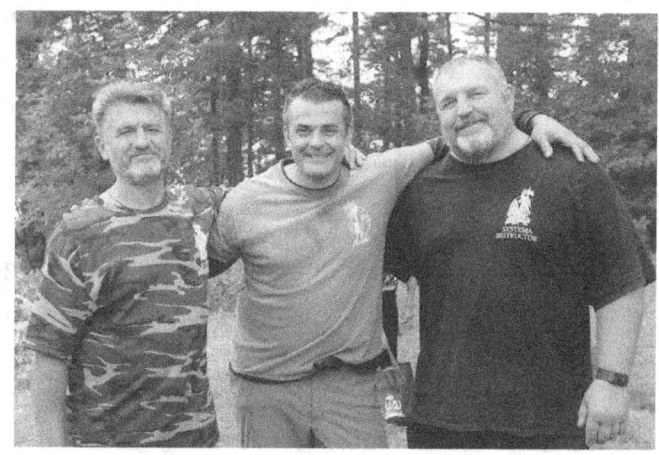

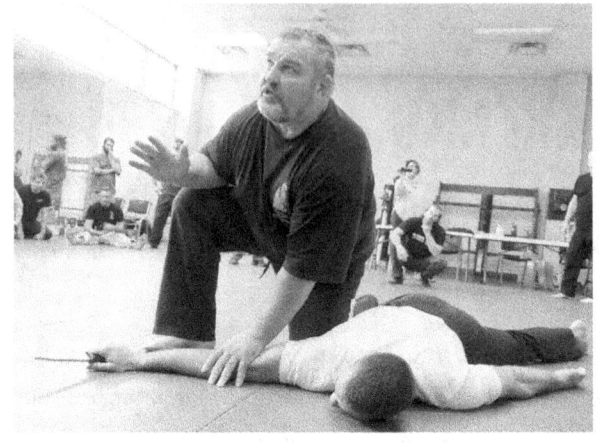

bars until black belt, for example, or practice chokes until you were 14. In my hometown we were taught and practiced those things since day one.

That's a very different approach, a different cultural background?

Yes, we did not have that litigation culture back home. Do you know of any Judo school, for example, that told you never to tap out from a choke? You either get out or pass out! That's how our coach was.

When did you first become aware of Systema and what were your first impressions?

At college I was lucky, one of the official Sombo founders was teaching there, so my Sombo coaches were his students. It was an original Sombo school, but I always felt that something was missing. It was a lot of techniques but there was no unifying idea behind it. Like making a salad without a plan or a recipe! I was talking to many people and some told me that this was actually filtered and watered down from the original Sombo and there were only about fifteen to twenty people left in the country who knew the original teachings. Later on, I found out that Mikhail was teaching just a few blocks from my college and I never knew about it. I actually found out about Systema when I moved to the States.

When was that?

That was about 1992. In 1993 I started teaching Judo and I first met Vladimir in 2003. So for around ten years I was teaching Judo in the States. I saw some of Vladimir's clips, then I met him at one of the Aiki Expos in Vegas. I didn't go there to see Vladimir, to be honest I thought all the clips I had seen looked fake. I couldn't take it seriously. I went to the Expo to try some Aikido, saw that this Russian guy was also there, so I thought I may as well drop in to see this nonsense. Vladimir's seminar was the first one and within about five minutes I realised that whatever it was I had been looking for, I had found. So Aikido was no longer on the list!

This seems to be a very common experience amongst Systema people!

Exactly, because when you know what are looking for, when you experience it you know what it is. It was interesting because I hadn't expected to find it, so I was very fortunate. Systema is very unifying, everything you can do is unified within one art, if you can call it art. I think the original name for it was "Know Thyself", which is a little more accurate. More difficult to market, perhaps.

So you had Mikhail right at home but had to travel to find Systema!

I had to go across the ocean to find it, yes! I met Mikhail later, when he came to the States. At that time Vladimir had already taken a few groups to Moscow. I joined just after that, I think he started in 1992, so had already been teaching for about ten years by that time.

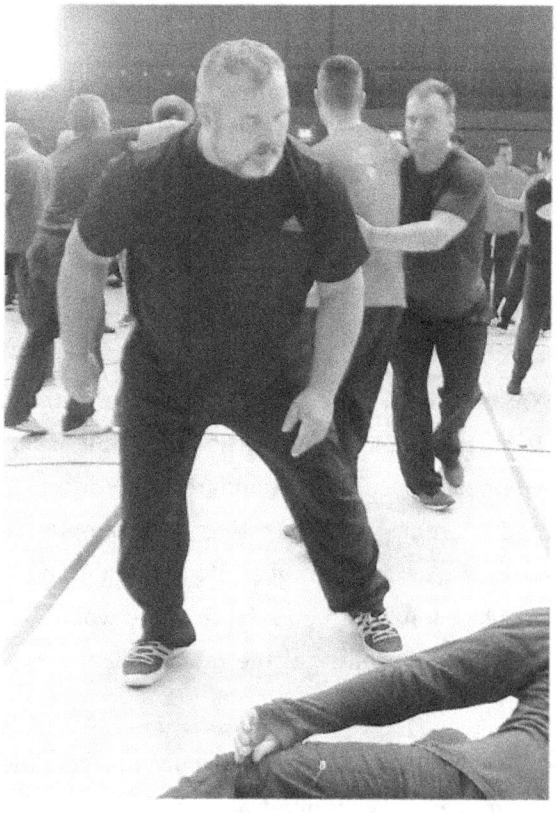

Does Judo still make up part of your training?

I was teaching for ten to twelve years, so both of my boys grew up doing Judo. My youngest began competing when he was five, at twelve he was National Champion. The older was just as good as

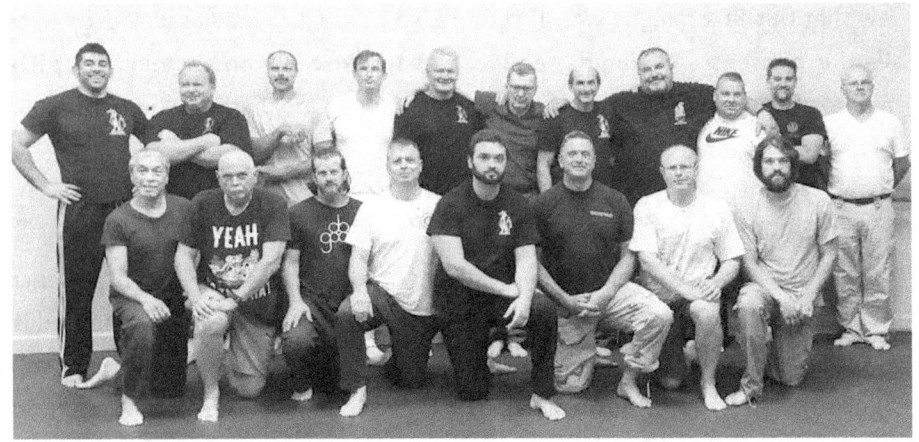

him. When I discovered Systema I could see the things that were wrong in what I was teaching them, so I began to fix things bit by bit. For a few years they were doing Systema in a Judo gi!

Do you think that in general competition is a good thing in martial arts?

Depends what you mean by "martial arts." Competition is a way you can test yourself in a sports setting. If the martial art is for combat there is no way you can do that.

How then do you think we can test our combat skills safely?

Well, if you want to really test you combat skills you have to get into combat. You cannot learn to swim without getting in the water! Back in the Karate times, some of the guys were testing themselves by getting into bar fights and the like. Not starting them but, if challenged, not backing down. Any competition assumes boundaries. Any sports martial art is formed by the rules and refereeing. Take wrestling, for example, back in ancient Greek times it was no rules, so it was combat. If you look at modern Olympic wrestling, it is very regulated. It has to be safe, or there would be no competition! Even the early UFC had less rules but there was still a referee to jump in and stop the fight before it was over.

Why do you think that so much entertainment, whether sports or other, still seems to revolve around violence?

Violence doesn't exist by itself, violence is a product of aggression, which is rooted in fear. I love martial arts but cannot watch MMA, when one is beating the other while he is on the ground, for example. But it pleases the crowd, it's like gladiators I imagine. In that sense our society is not developing, we are going backwards. Even slavery is back, in another form, debt is economic slavery!

Do you see Systema as an antidote to some of those negative influences?

Well, whatever is happening in society, you can only change yourself, to start. From there you may have a chance to help someone else on the way. From a religious view, the saying is that saving your soul is your main priority. If you save yourself you can then perhaps help save someone else.

So you had been teaching Judo already, when did you start teaching Systema and was it very different?

It gave me a different view on what I had previously been doing, how much better I could be training, how much safer the training could be. In a way you can practice Systema in any art. For example, you can be training in BJJ but be doing Systema without people knowing. You are doing the breathing, you find your way to move, to survive. Systema is universal, very adaptable, it's not even a martial art. I think people start it as a martial art then realise it is much bigger. Everyone you talk to who has been doing Systema for more than a couple of years will tell you that whatever their original goal was, it has now changed. The value becomes much greater than was

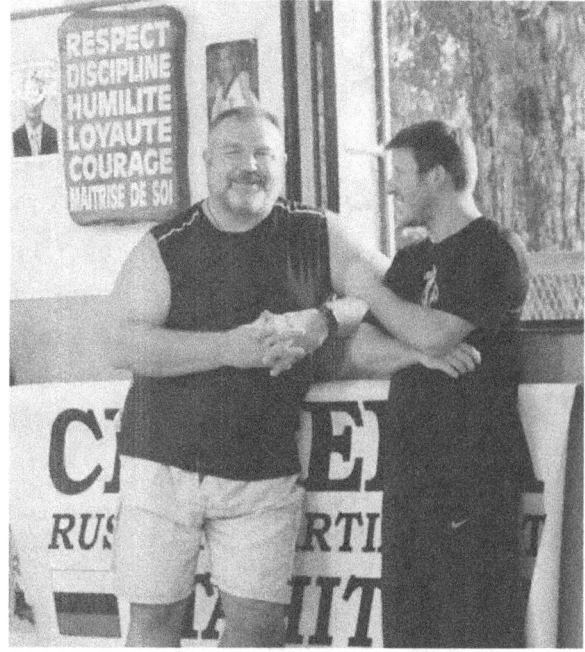

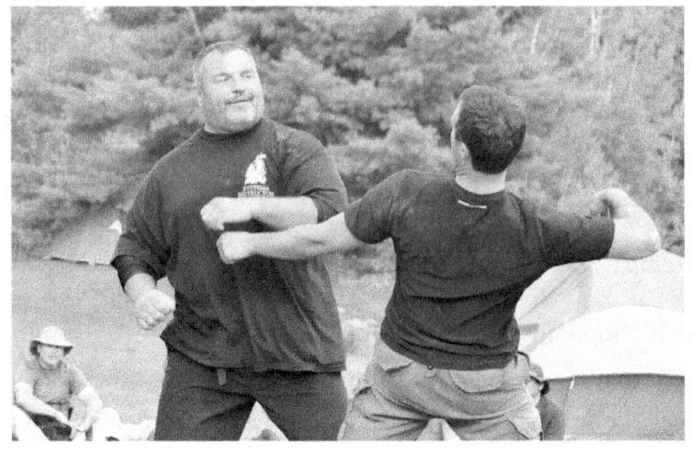

originally thought. *Do you find that people from different backgrounds are coming into Systema now?*

I teach regular seminars and one that I teach every three months is on breath and bodywork. I have more participation, I have more interest in that one than any other subject. It's not combative in any way, we do five hours of massage, breath work, bettering yourself, helping your partner. Last time I did it the age range was from eight to eighty-five! Everyone was on the mat, everyone was doing the same work, all enjoying themselves. In the circle up at the end everyone made good comments. What could be better?

What do you think of martial arts as a business? Are things more commercial these days?

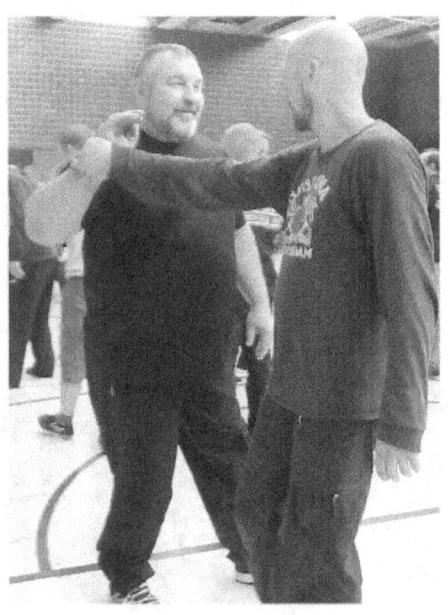

In the States the business of the martial arts is really dictated by what is popular in MMA. So at the moment that's Thai Boxing and BJJ. Probably BJJ more, because it is less traumatic. If you remember, the original BJJ from the Gracie family was pretty rudimentary compared to what you see now. There were no leg locks, very limited grab work. Now, they have leg locks, they have added many things in, so it is the biggest growing martial art right now. But I expect it will decline. As the rules start changing, the art starts to change.

As a sport I think BJJ is fantastic. In Systema we spend less time on the ground as we have different priorities. In BJJ they spend less time recovering from the intense work they do, which is a deficiency. But commercially BJJ is doing very well. I'm glad that Systema is not that commercialised. If you start changing it in order to sell it, then it is no longer the original product.

Do you think that makes it difficult to run a Systema school as a business?

There are people doing it, but it is very difficult, I think. To

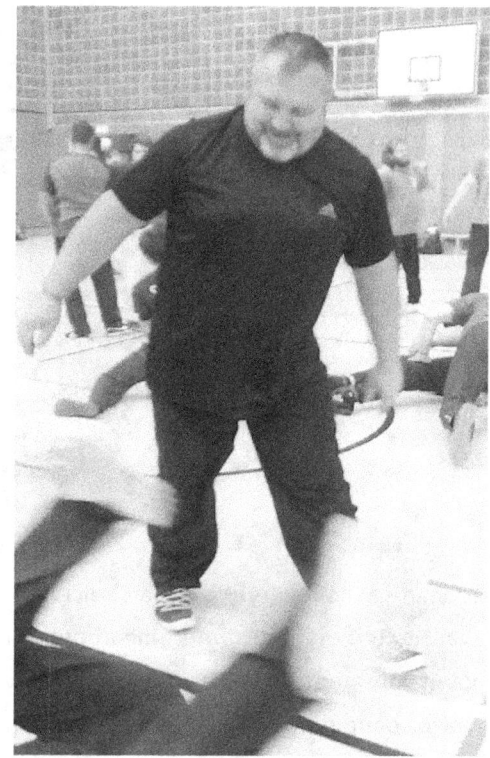

maintain the balance between the art and the commercial aspect is tough. I prefer not to do that, I prefer not to make a living from Systema, it takes away that complication for me. I can teach exactly how and what I want to.

What do you do for a living?

I'm a professional bureaucrat!

So you always have work?

Yes, I have job security (laughs)

How do you think that Systema should be promoted, given that these days you have to have some form of promotion?

I think the way Vladimir and Valerie have been doing it for years is the best way. They have a great sense of how not to under or over promote, it's hard to think how it could be done better. There is no degrading of other arts, they

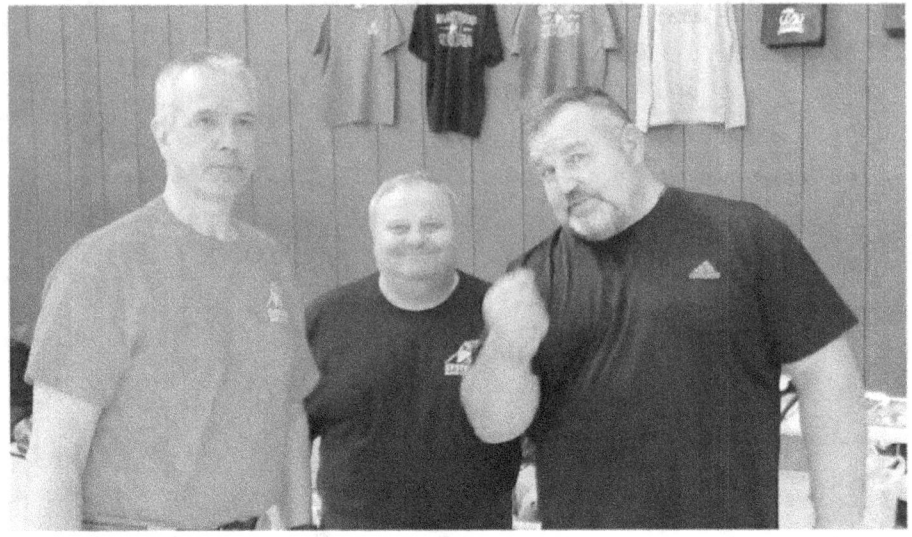

recognise that everyone has a choice. And when it comes to Systema, if people want to understand something about it, they need to try it. Because you see a lot of comments from people who never will. So their comments have no value, but of course on the screen those comments count as much as those of the people who talk from experience. That's why I have great respect for people who come to train for the first time. They have decided to bite the bullet and try something they have not done before. At an event like this, they can train with so many different people as well as the Masters, of course.

And mix with people from all over the world.

Yes, no one cares where you are from. Systema helps keep an even relationship between people. None of us is perfect, as humans we all screw up. But I think the community we have helps keep people morally healthier. Systema helps you to liberate yourself from your fears and it is the fears in your life that make you do ugly things. The less fear we have, the more pure and human we can be. Then we can enjoy life!

Have there been any particular circumstances where Systema has helped you through?

I got sick a few years back, my spine got infected and I became paralysed. I spent about a month in hospital, mostly in an ICU. Following that I had to learn how to walk all over again. The pain I endured was quite overwhelming but I decide not to rely on drugs. Instead I went into the Systema breath work and that was my salvation.

I had a physical therapist come to the house, but within a couple of sessions she realised that I was teaching her more than she was showing me! She did help with massage and getting special equipment for me, though. But I owe my recovery to Systema and am lucky in many ways because of it.

Such a simple thing as breathing!

Well it can get very involved, when you see what Mikhail can do and we cannot! But breathing is a rabbit hole, you see how much further it goes from a simple start. You never master it. I've not seen anyone who has found the end of the hole yet. If you find it, let me know!

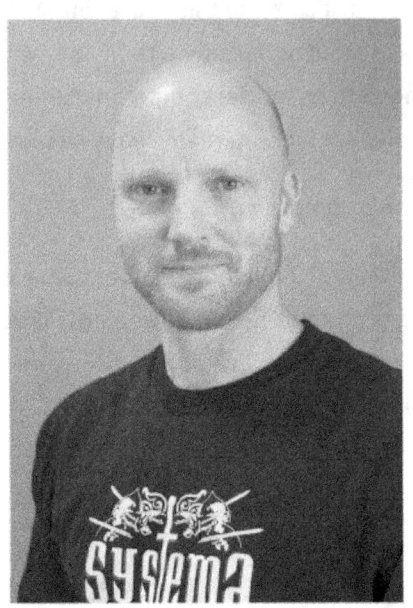

GLENN MURPHY

Can you first tell us something of your background?

I was born and raised in Kent, England, on the south coast. I moved up to Scotland to attend University, in Aberdeen. I was studying genetics and immunology and it was there that I also started studying martial arts seriously. After that, I moved to Japan for a couple of years, where I met my wife, then moved back to live in London. In 2007 we moved to the US, North Carolina, and have lived here ever since, with our two kids. I used to run operations at the Learning Department at the Museum of Science and Industry in London, when I left there I started writing popular science books. I've written 25 now, they are aimed at high school level kids. Nowadays I also teach Systema and run corporate training on stress, health and personal protection.

What was it that first got you into martial arts?

My family were always very sporty. My dad was actually a professional soccer player, mostly for Second Division teams in Kent, and a couple of times for Ipswich and Chelsea. But he got a bad knee injury that took him out of the professional level. We actually lived just behind a sports centre in Folkestone, so as kids we would always be going swimming, playing tennis and the like. I played soccer but it was clear I was never going to be that good at it, I was better at kicking

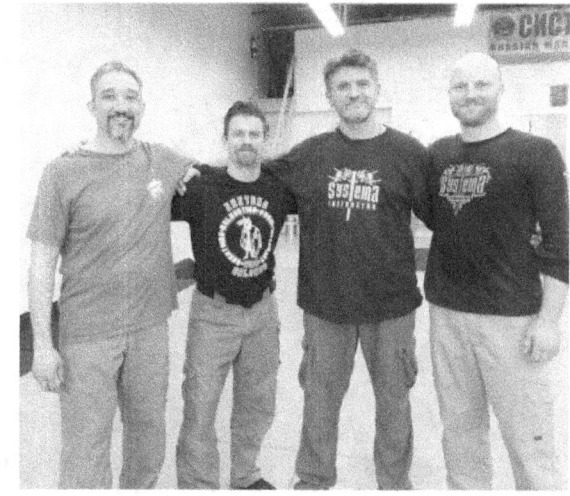

other players than the ball (laughs). So I guess I channelled that into martial arts, starting with Judo when I was about seven. I didn't do that for very long, I soon moved on to Karate for a while. I also took up Fencing, I competed in that while at school. I tried a couple of other things too, such as Bujinkan Ninjitsu. At University there was a very strong Aikido club, set up by a guy called Gerry Hinton, who had spent a lot of years in Japan training with Morohito Seito.

And you travelled to Japan yourself?

Yes, after Uni I went to Japan for two years to train at the Owama Dojo. As well as training I wanted some time out to decide what I was going to do after my degree. Eventually, I decided to continue my science education, so came back to London to study Science Communication at the Imperial College.

Did you begin teaching Aikido when you came back to London?

I did, yes, initially at the Science Museum. I started dabbling in other stuff too, Escrima, Kali, some Taiji and Bagua. I was very interested in the underpinning of Aikido, where did it come from? There's a Ju Jitsu root, of course, but also a definite pre-war and post-war version. It seems that the founder, Ueshiba, was very much influenced by his time in Manchuria and is said to have studied from Bagua teachers there. So it was interesting to study Bagua from that perspective, though I never achieved any real proficiency in it.

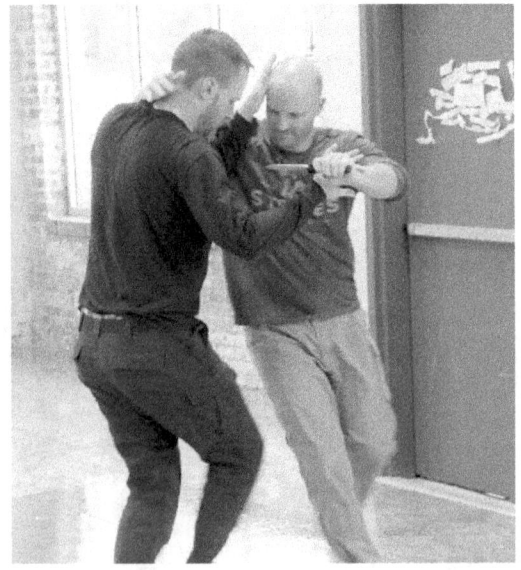

And when did you first hear about Systema?

While I was at the Imperial College I saw a flier from a guy called Sam Benson, who was teaching a group just by the college. I think I may have already seen a couple of VHS tapes, which got me curious, so

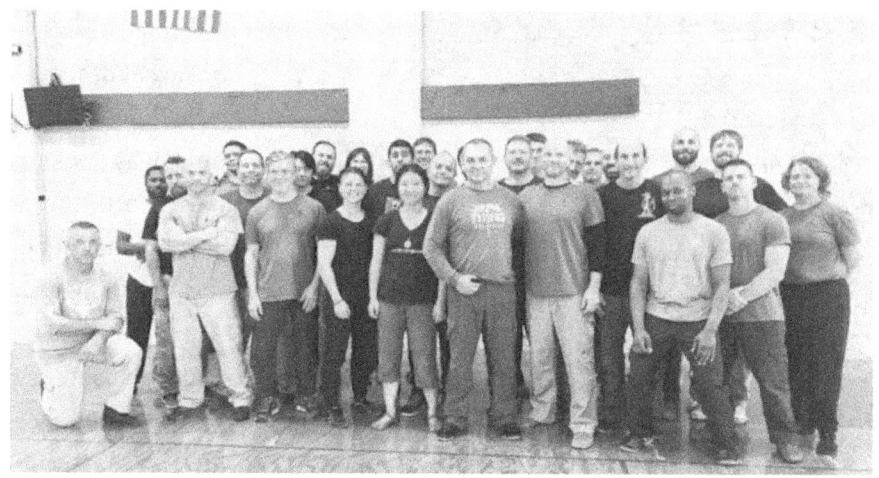

I thought I'd try Sam's class. I was very impressed with his skill and also the attitude of the people training.

And how did this affect your Aikido?

Having put so many years into it, I was very reluctant to let go of the Aikido. So I trained both for a while but eventually realised the only reason I was still doing the Aikido was because I felt confident and competent in it! I pretty much dropped it when I moved to the US and began training in North Carolina. In fact, I met Vladimir two months later, and that was it!

So your first exposure was the old video tapes?

Yes and I thought it looked cool, so I tried to mimic the techniques but nothing was working! Of course, I had no foundation. One thing that really impressed me at Sam's class, the first day I went, they were doing counter-throws. It was on a wooden floor and I thought surely someone would get injured but everyone was hitting the ground softly. I tried applying some locks on Sam but he just dissolved out of them, it was very disconcerting that he escaped everything in way that wasn't obvious to me. It was clear that the understanding of bio-mechanics was way ahead of mine. Then I tried taking and giving hits, which I also struggled with. It was a big kick in the ego.

Did you think that this was what you had been looking for in martial arts?

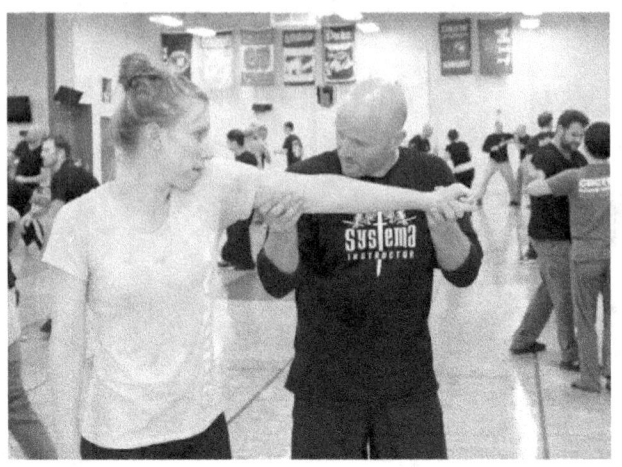

Well I was still looking at other things at the time. I think, for me I was looking at martial arts that had all the usual benefits, plus perhaps some kind of lifestyle approach too. So with Aikido I got immersed into the whole culture of it but I began to feel I was pretending to be Japanese, it was all a bit alien still. Systema didn't do that, it just asked you to be your own person. I think once I realised that what was Systema was about, I jumped ship wholesale.

And what prompted the move to the States?

My wife is American. Her dad was in the military, so she moved around a lot but her family were still in the States. Also, as by then I was writing, I could work from pretty much anywhere. It was good luck that two months after I moved here, Mark Jacobson, who teaches in Charlotte, NC, brought Vladimir down for a two day seminar. So that was my first meeting with Vladimir and also the first time I'd trained Systema for longer than an hour and a half! It was two days on multiple attackers. We were working in groups of six, two stood back to back and the other four attacked. I was covered in bruises by the end, it was great (laughs). Seeing how Vladimir moved was fantastic too. Plus I met three people there from my part of NC, so we formed a training group when we got back.

Is that when you started teaching?

At first it was more just the group of us training. But a year later I went up to the Toronto Camp and managed to become an Instructor in Training. When I came back I had stronger fundamentals and some good tools, so I started leading the group. It took about another year or two before I went full time with the teaching.

And in the early days, how did you structure your classes?

The very early days I just copied the progressions on the video. We would basically try and copy what we saw on the DVDs, which was okay as a start. Then I began to mix up ideas a little bit, especially after going to the Camp. Konstantin, in particular, was very helpful, he set out different themes day by day. So the first day was contact, we focussed on rolling, getting used to contact on the body. The second day was precision, we did nothing but touch with fists and feet. Then we did a whole day on knives, then power, then onto strikes.

So he set out this whole process, this hierarchy, which, of course, he later put into his book too. Beginning with motivation, then building the combative body, followed by the psyche. From there into movement, then to wrestling, striking, working with weapons and so on. Once I had that I felt I had a framework to build my own training progressions.

Who else has influenced your teaching style?

Oh, Emmanuel Manolakais, without a doubt. I've trained with him a lot. Specifically, there was one book he recommended to me, which changed my perception of how people learn and how to teach. So in the early days I'd map out a class plan but now I tend to go in with a theme and see how things develop, where people are, what the feeling in the room is and I'll start to adjust. I may still have a specific goal sometimes but it's not so fixed as before. The important thing is that everyone leaves feeling energised and happy.

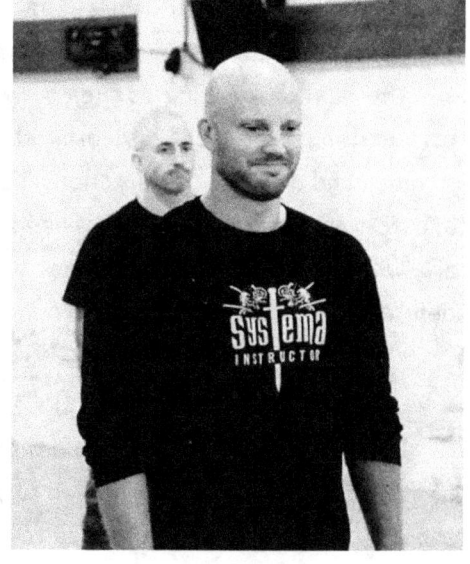

Do you find Systema gives you the tools to be creative and spontaneous? And does that cross over into other aspects of life?

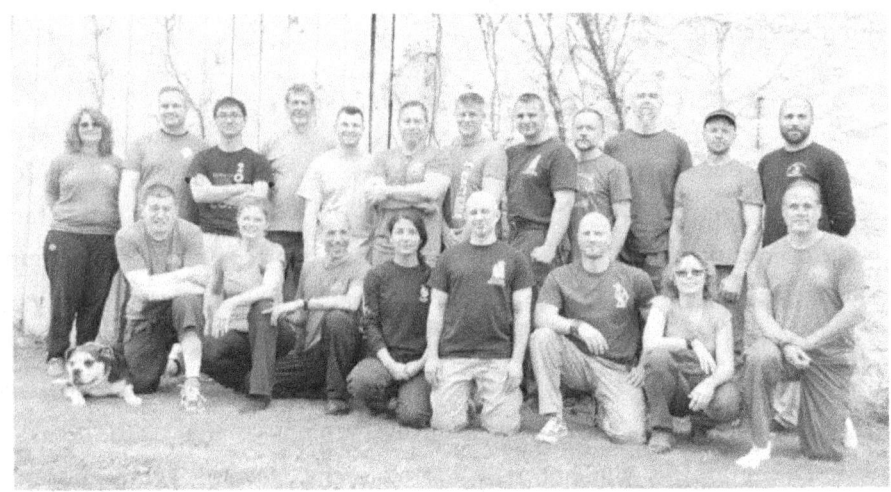

That's a good question. I think I've always been good at assimilating information, I'm a voracious reader. I can pick a lot of things up, then integrate them into a format that sounds like my own. So it sounds like I'm improvising but I'm actually translating other people's ideas. I guess in one sense, there is nothing new and all art is theft but I think Systema has made me a lot more creative. Even in something like playing guitar. I've been playing guitar since I was twelve but again, copying other people's solos. Even the improvisation was a copy of someone else. It's only in recent years that I've genuinely really enjoyed being totally spontaneous when playing, really enjoying each note, getting a bit more Miles Davies! That purely comes from Systema, before, I couldn't do that for the fear of sounding bad somehow.

The same in writing as well , I was quite derivative before, basically restructuring someone else's work with a little of my own. Now, I'm not writing so much and do more presentations, but I find I'm really enjoying the creation of a story and a narrative. Systema has developed my ability to see where people are, where they need to be and how to get them there. I wasn't truly creative before, it's just been this past five or six years.

How big a role is removing or managing fear in that process?

I think it's central to the whole thing. The fear not just of failing but what of others will think, of not living up to your full potential... there are so many aspects of our daily lives governed to a greater extent than we would like to admit by our innate fears. Some we learn growing up, some are taught by parents, some come from formative experiences. Letting go of those fears is a wonderfully liberating experience. You realise there is so much you are capable of. But it's a process, right? We can't always see just how afraid of failure or other things we are, but when we train Systema it reminds us on a daily level to let go of that fear. That gives you a new capacity to be able to create without fear of messing it up all the time. You start to embrace failure as a lesson in itself, to use it is a guide for the future.

There's a lot of intellectual understanding around of that, I mean in the business world they say, "Don't be afraid to make mistakes" but they don't actually want you to make mistakes! The real paradigm shift with Systema is that you have to make mistakes in order to figure out where your shortcomings are. In a way, you seek out your weaknesses, then you find new depths to work with. Admitting you have fear is the first step, not masking it. Then you can look at the reasons as to why you might have it, where you developed it, why you hold onto it, then start to let that go. It's a huge topic.

In your experience, is there a difference in being an instructor in Systema and an instructor in another style?

I think there are the same risks when it comes to attitude. Being a Systema instructor doesn't make us immune to the possibility of becoming egotistical, for example. The very fact that the methodology encourages humility and encourages us to be self aware inoculates us to a certain extent. As long as you continue training with the top teachers and getting that humility and reality check, then you're in a lot less danger than maybe if you are a "big master" who rests on their laurels. So that helps, you have to keep checking

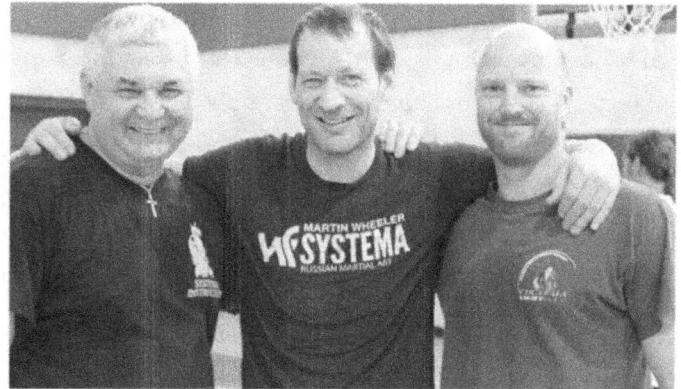

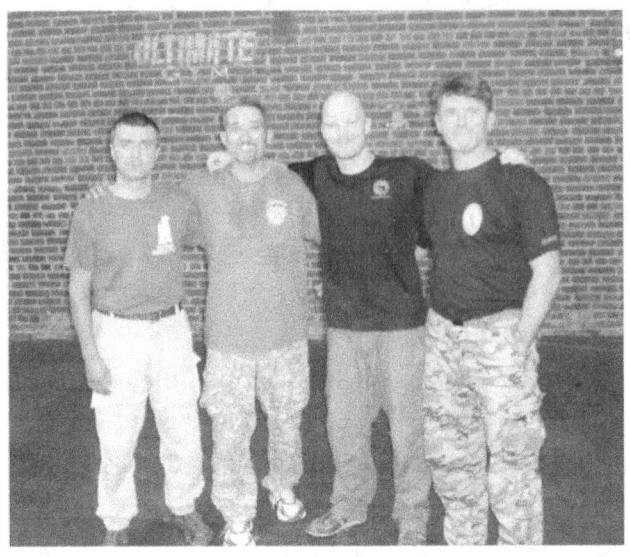

in, that's the key thing. I also the think the fact that Systema instructors get involved in the training helps, too. Not just dishing out but being on the receiving end as well.

I remember in my Aikido days, the teacher would watch us train, then intermittently come in and demonstrate a couple of techniques, but in a safe, controlled environment. Of course under those conditions, everything looks great. And I'm not saying he wasn't capable, because he was. But there is a huge vulnerability to what we do as instructors in Systema, because we work with students as though we are students ourselves. We open ourselves up to fail and we often do, but showing that vulnerability is key. I think people respect that. Other styles can rest on a hierarchy, or you have to attack in a certain way, it becomes something not quite real.

Do you find that approach also attracts more professionals?

Well yes, there's a lot of military guys train with us, very experienced, such as my friend Tommy, he's a former Green Beret. Those guys are not easily convinced by anything, right? If you just talk a good game, tell them how good you are, recite your lineage, it means absolutely nothing to these guys. All they care about is what skills do you have and can you transfer them to me? Those guys appreciate right away that you are touching hands with them, you are striking them and letting them strike you. They see the integrity in that and that is a rare thing in martial arts. I'm not saying it's unique to Systema but I think it is uncommon in a lot of other arts.

As instructors we all have types of work that we like more than others. How do you balance showing what are good at, with what you are not so good at?

I guess the simple answer to that is very poorly (laughs). I think we are constantly developing. I was talking to Brad Scornavacco recently, we were talking about how there are three sets of skills as a Systema instructor. One is your ability as a Systema practitioner. Second is how you are as a teacher, your ability to transmit knowledge. Third is the ability in getting people to come to your classes, the business skills, if you like. Those are completely independent things, you may be great at one but suck at another, right? So you have to work on your ability to teach as much as your ability to do. So if I just taught the things I'm good at, maybe my students would get okay too but they would be missing out on all the things I'm subconsciously filtering out.

For example, if I didn't like ground work and never really showed it much, then the students are denied the capacity not only to develop their ground work but also to see the connections between working on the ground and stand up. How the relaxation of spine and hips carries over between the two, for example. Or the relationships in grappling you can use when standing, or the skills that cross over into your striking work. They'll lose that whole vocabulary if you are selfish in your teaching. That's one aspect. The other thing is as a student myself, I think I would stagnate if I just continued to work on the things I'm good at and avoid the things I'm bad at. In teaching terms, it's a difficult thing. What I've tried to do over the years is continue to add in any work I get from when I train at HQ.

Because I may be there for nine days and learn some new drills and exercises, but it takes time for all of that knowledge to settle and consolidate. So that's usually the thing I'll focus on for the next

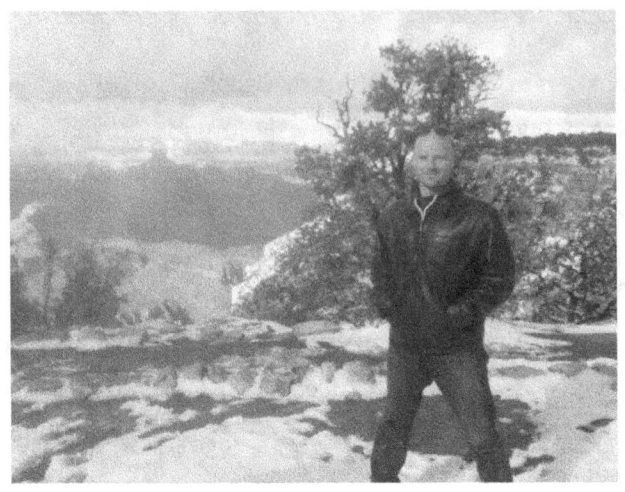

couple of months of teaching, because now I have some more understanding of it, or see it from different angles.

I used to avoid teaching things that I only had a tenuous grasp on but then I thought if I don't do that, I'd never be working on those things. So in a way, teaching those things forces me to work on them, too. The balance is then to give the basic parameters of the drill and let people work on it at a foundational level but try not to over explain it verbally and to let people know this is something we are trying out. That has also made me less afraid of trying things with the group that I have less experience of myself.

You mentioned verbal explanation there. Was there any conflict with your background as a science writer and teaching an art which is, when it comes down to it, formless?

It was a big problem at the beginning. I was trying to see Systema through the lens of the other arts I'd done, particularly Aikido. So every time I saw I movement I'd say, "Oh, that's irimi nage," for example, rather than taking it on its own value. That was something that took a few years to let go of. The deeper tendency, to want to break things down into parts, to be reductionist, the scientific approach in its sense of take it all apart, examine every piece in minute detail, then try and put it all back together again... I found in Systema that is counter-productive. But it has taken me a long time to let go of, even now I sometimes still try and analyse like it was a machine. So you can analyse bio-mechanics, yes, you get a deeper understanding of bio-mechanics, which, to a certain extent is necessary. After all you need to know about leverage, about centre of mass, about balance and good form and so on, though you don't have to know the names of each minor body part.

What I do is sprinkle bits of that into the training, particularly if people are struggling with something. So I might talk about patterns of tension in the body, perhaps relate it to two sets of pulleys in the body, things like that. The problem with over-analysing bio-mechanics is that you get a good understanding of two static systems and move them around as if they are robots. But we are not working with dummies, we are working with a living, breathing organism that has fears and desires. Those things are what we primarily act from, not from bio-mechanics.

That's not to say you can't do a very good bio-mechanical breakdown that's hard to resist. You can but it will never be exactly the same twice, because the people you are working with a different shapes and sizes, they will have different intrinsic flinch responses to the things you are trying to apply to them. Even the top MMA guys who can apply explosive take downs, well, if you are quick and see it coming, it doesn't work. So people try and get round that by moving as fast as possible, or by throwing some kind of feint first. In Systema, instead, we acknowledge that every person has a switched on nervous system, so we try and work in a way that slips past the nervous system, to be smooth and non-threatening.

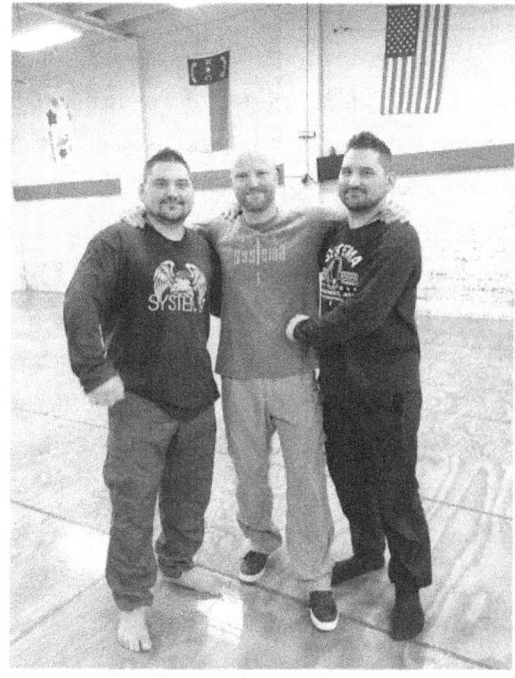

If you are constantly tied up with the idea of bio-mechanics, then you miss this whole other world of neurology and psychology, and what Vladimir calls the "real power" that comes from it. Bio-mechanics is a fundamental, a building block, certainly, but not something to become obsessed with.

I guess the same applies to any aspect of training?

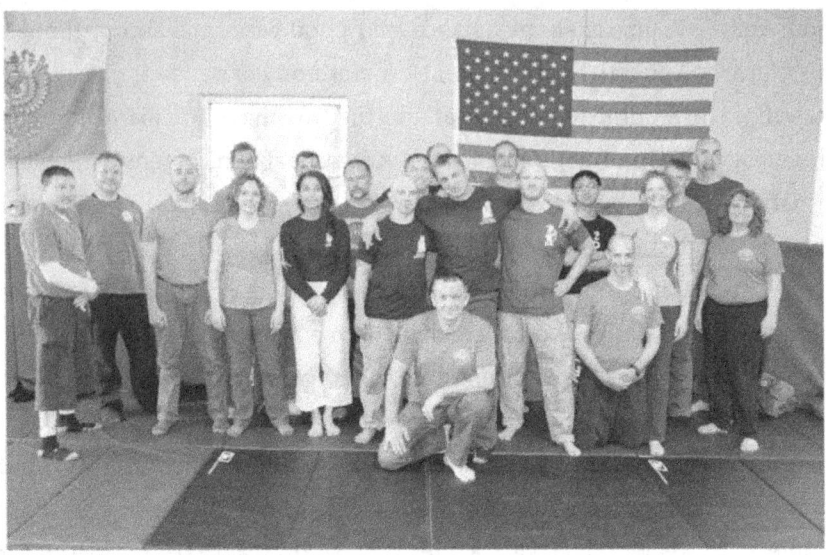

Yes, so you may get obsessed with wave energy, or psychological work or similar, you may try it but have terrible physical form. There has to be a balance there. Now, rather than reduce, I find it is more about trying to recapture the state I had when it was working, to take a snapshot of that instant.

Does that mean the way you train has changed a lot?

Yes, well for one thing my motivations changed. In the beginning the training was to help me be more effective in martial arts. The Aikido was useful in certain realms but I couldn't move so well on the ground, or work against weapons and so on. I was looking to fill in the gaps, I guess. When I started training Systema properly, I realised that even the things I thought I could do, I couldn't actually do that well (laughs). So for a few years after that it was a quest to try and gain some basic competency. Then it became a fascination with learning the art itself. That first Immersion Camp, the state I came back home in, after training in the forest and all the rest of it... I was a different person, psychologically. More calm, happier, more resilient. So then I thought, this is it, this is what I want more of. If you can be as strong as you can as a person, then people can lean hard on you and you can do good things in life. That's why I train now, to be honest. There's a lot of stress in life, that is inevitable, so the quest to become stronger and be able to stay calmer is important. To be a good dad, to be a good husband, be a good teacher, to help other people, all those things.

Systema was like a mirror, for me, it showed me all things I thought were strengths were actually weaknesses. I was arrogant, full of pride. It showed me that the more I can clean myself psychologically, the more I can help others. That's been the thread that's carried me through the last ten years of training.

I believe you've started a Systema podcast?

Yes, partly because I wanted to proselytise a bit, to show that Systema is not just a martial art you learn for combat. It's been very enjoyable, I get to speak to people with more experience than me and pilfer their insight (laughs). It's been great to get so many perspectives, some that agree with your own and others that contradict. There's a great pool of knowledge gathered over the last few years in the Systema community, I really wanted to open that up on a global level.

The idea really came from not being able to explain what Systema was when people asked! Some see or promote it from the tough military angle, no belts, no nonsense. But there is this dissonance between that form of advertising and what actually happens when people come to class, right? If you advertise that way, you may attract a certain type of person and then they may be disappointed when you have them doing breath work for half an hour. On the flip side, others may look at that type of advertising and think it is not for them at all. Those are the people I was more interested in attracting, the people who don't understand it has this whole mind-body capacity. There's a whole new fascination now with people

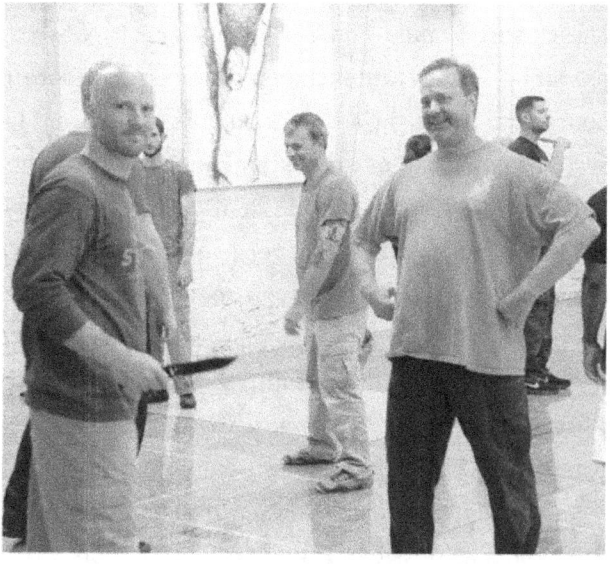

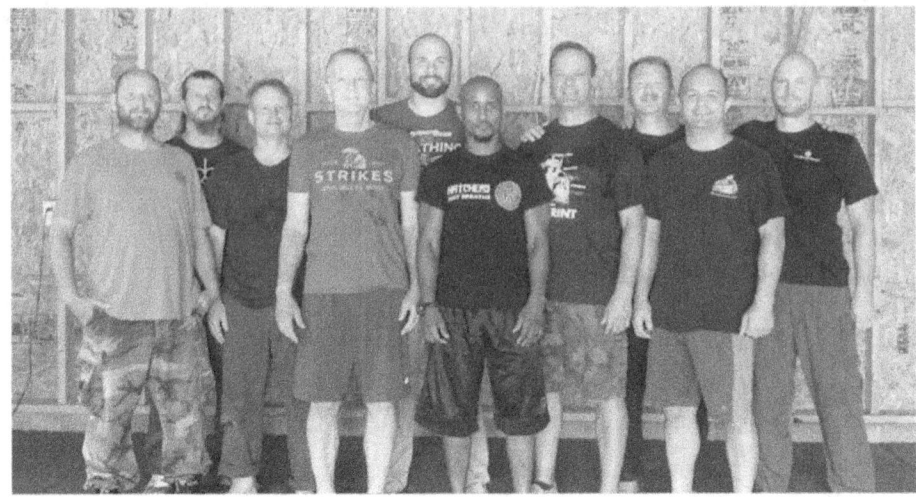

studying movement for its own benefits. Those people would love Systema but why are they not coming? So I thought how can I re-frame this, to capture the martial essence that Systema has to offer, not to tone it down to "moving Yoga", but to pitch it in such a way that a person interested in movement, stress control, in survival, how could I reach all of those people?

So how do you explain Systema and how have you promoted your classes?

If you tell people that Systema can achieve all these things, they don't believe you. They say, no you have to do twelve things to achieve all that, right? The closest I could come to explaining it, was to describe Systema as an operating system rather than a style. So that became my main driver for the podcast, to talk to different instructors, at different levels. I ask how they found Systema, which helps understand how others can find it, what is their concept of it, to get different facets and also how it applies to wider life. That's why I called the podcast Systema for Life, to put across this idea that the primary benefit from training is that you apply it to your wider life. It infuses the rest of your life and makes it better.

Now you can say the same thing about Yoga or Tai Chi to an extent but Systema is not only in that same field, it is more powerful in its effect. Because you learn to work under pressure, not just when you are relaxed and in a nice environment. So I really wanted to emphasise that and get as many different viewpoints as possible. I thought I'd give it six months, but here we are nine months in, with ten thousand regular listeners and a lot of nice feedback from the Systema community.

Do you think that Systema is evolving?

Very much so. If you look back at the work put out by HQ, initially it was very much about physical movement, about articulating individual joints of the body. That developed into strengthening the core, then there was a big emphasis on breathing. Not just burst breathing to recover but how breathing drives everything. Not just your movement but your decisions, the way that you move. More recently it's about relaxed power. So the things that come down the pipeline are changing, it is definitely evolving. That is something else that sets it apart from the traditional disciplines. There, the emphasis is on passing things down unchanged, so lineage becomes very important. Now in Systema it is good, of course, to train with the top teachers, but the point is they are not just giving out static knowledge, they aren't holding little bits back to keep you in place. Their understanding is evolving as well, and they pass that change down the line. There's no veneer of authority, it's all very open.

Any final thoughts you'd like to share?

I've been in a fortunate place, where I've got to enjoy confluence of having the ability to teach very well with being exposed to people who have really great skill. I try not to pass on my mistakes, I try and translate what I learn from others with as much fidelity as I can. As an instructor, if you can learn and teach with integrity I don't think you can go too far wrong. Be honest about what you can and can't do and check in often! It's so risky to go off on your own musings and interpretations for too long. I think we need to see the top teachers at least once or twice a year, to get that reality check on what we think we know. That's probably the single most valuable thing you can do.

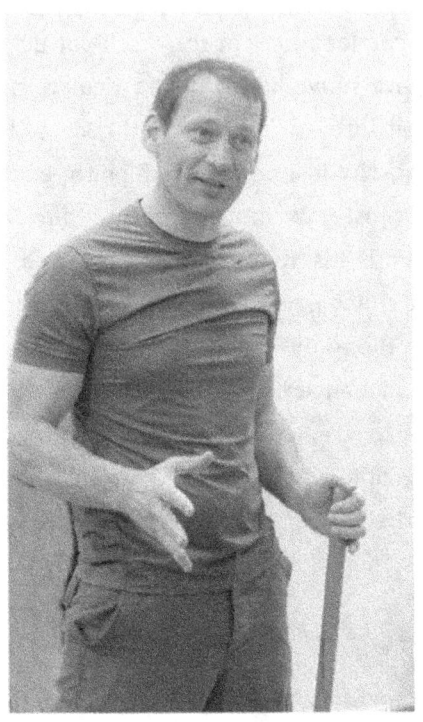

MARTIN WHEELER

Perhaps we could start with something about your background? Where you are from, how did you get into martial arts and so on.

In terms of martial arts, the first thing I remember watching was the Kung Fu TV series. As far as training goes, my friends and I went to a Judo club when I was about 8, they kind of fell away but I stuck with it. At about 15 I started training in Ed Parker's Kenpo Karate, there was a local club in my hometown. The club was known as the Doormans Academy, it's where all the local door guys trained. I was brought up in a small town, a south of England holiday resort. In the summer it was always busy with people on holiday or people coming down for the weekend, so there were lots of fights. In the winter there was no work so people would get drunk and fight each other (laughs).

It was a very good Kenpo club, I learned a lot there. It was a lot of bare knuckle sparring, I was training with adults. It's good training when you are young but I don't think you can keep doing it!

Kenpo must have been quite rare in the UK at the time?

Yes, apart from in the South West, I believe, there was no other Kenpo in the whole of the UK. There was Karate and Judo but Kenpo was rare – that was good though because it meant the quality was high. Gary Ellise and Bob Rose had four clubs running, the guys were teaching what they knew and what they were using.

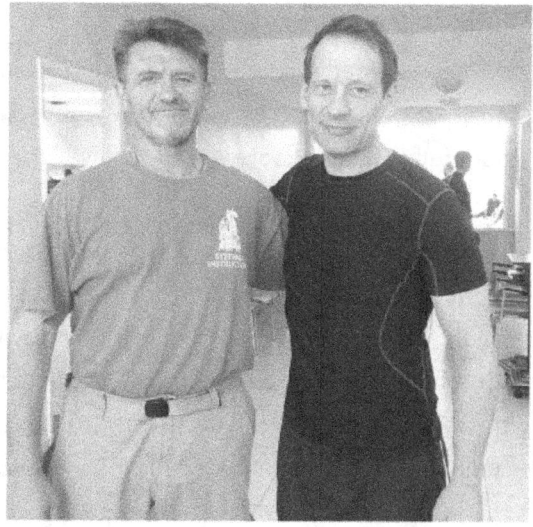

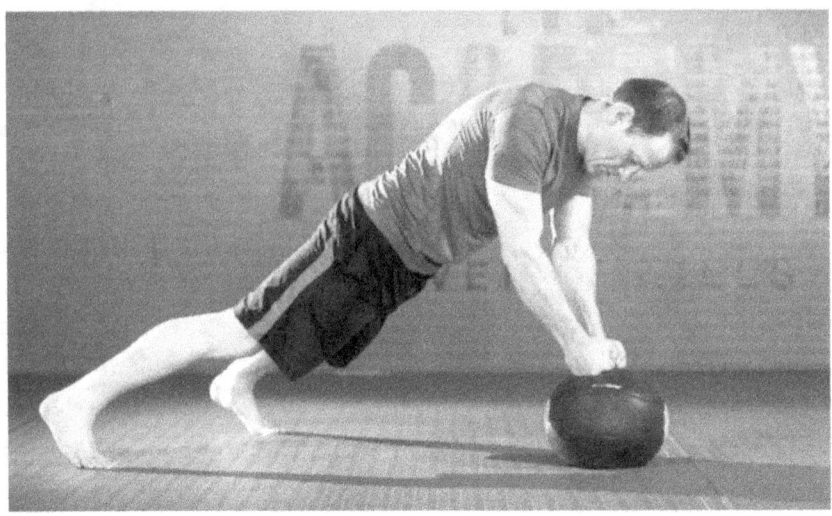

Did you ever meet Ed Parker?

Yes, quite a few times. He was a very enigmatic guy, it was quite a system he had. Kenpo is a very good system, it's misunderstood a lot. Some of the training methods are dated, but Ed Parker had a very modern concept of an art. I shifted into boxing, Thai boxing and back into Judo as well, because I knew Ed Parker had done those things too. I figured they would help me understand Kenpo better and it did, those arts helped a lot. I was a bouncer for ten years which of course is an education too!

So you had quite a rounded experience before you came to Systema?

Yes. I trained in some Filipino styles too with Huk Planas, he was Ed Parker's right hand man. Between them they put together this good mix of things, a good, full contact system.

What was your first exposure to Systema, was it through Vladimir?

No, actually it was through a friend of mine Al McLuckie, a well-known Filipino / Kenpo guy. He'd been training with Vladimir for about a year but didn't tell me about it. He kept coming up with these different things. I'd say, "this is brilliant, I love this stuff". Then later I went to a seminar in Florida that Vladimir had been invited to teach at. After about five seconds of watching him work I could see, "ah, that's the stuff" (laughs). I'd never seen anything like it. So I started training with Vladimir. I was living in Kentucky at the time and used to drive up. The first week of training with him blew away everything I knew. I tried everything and ended up in a lot of bad positions!

So that must have been in the early days of the Toronto school?

Yes it must have been 18 years ago. It was a different school back then – not better or worse, but different. There were a lot of military guys there then, it had just started to change to more civilian-style training.

Did you find the Systema training was more about refining what you already had rather than learning a lot of new things?

At first, perhaps. You already have what you have, you know you can do certain things. When those cropped up in training I wasn't encouraged not to use them. But after a while you discover that if you want to understand Systema you have to let go of everything. You can re-introduce them later, but to really understand you have to let go. I still struggle with describing Systema as a martial art. Or perhaps it is a martial art and the other ones aren't! It's more of a human art, you can point it at anything you want, it just so happens we point it in a martial direction.

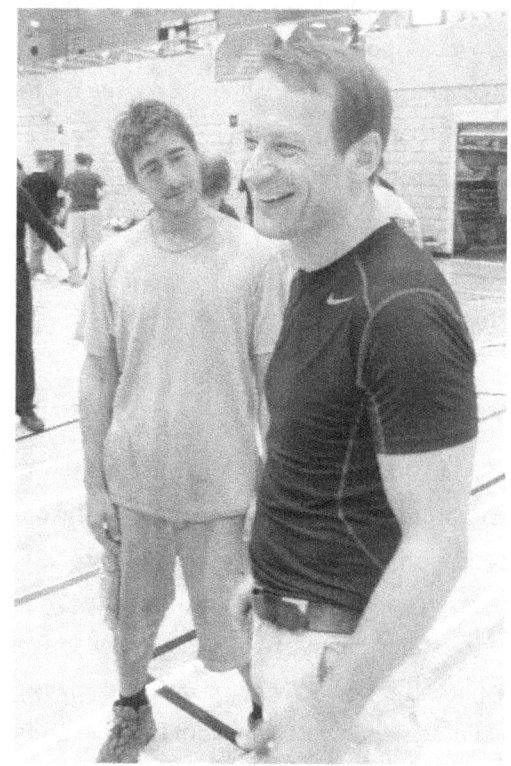

Do you find that makes it difficult to bring new people in though?

Well I don't think many people are looking for a "human art". They are looking for a

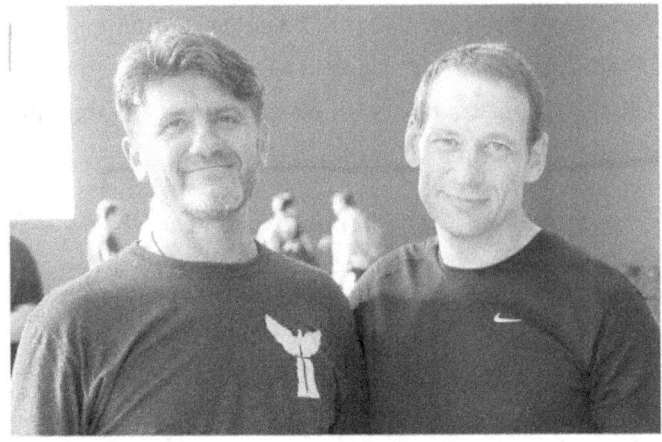

martial art and find something bigger when they come into this.

How did you get into teaching Systema? Were you already teaching in Kenpo?

Yes, I was doing seminars, travelling around the country with Kenpo. I'd been to New York teaching for a long time, they told me it was funny, one day I turned up and said, "Right, we're not doing that any more we're doing this!".

Did you encounter any resistance to the change?

I think there was some surprise, there'd been expectations of what I might do in Kenpo. There was one instructor who asked, "Don't you have any loyalty?" I told him that yes, I highly respected my teachers, but when it comes to training there's only one person I have loyalty to and that's me! It's a strange term, you can have loyalty to friends and teachers but it doesn't mean you have to train in the things they are doing.

What were your early experiences in Systema? Did you find it easier or more difficult to teach?

It was more fun! I was a little burned out teaching techniques. I was already teaching full contact stuff anyway, I was always interested in street application. So I just kind of transitioned it into the new approach... help people to relax, breathe, explore things a little more. Of course I had stumbling blocks teaching and learning, but it's all part of the process. Learning and teaching are in parallel – you can't learn without teaching it. You can't just go to a class and be taught Systema, you have to pass the knowledge on in order to understand it. Everyone thinks they know Systema until they have to explain it to someone else (laughs). People watch Systema from the side and they have one of three opinions –

1. That's amazing
2. That would never work, or
3. What are they doing!

You only really start to understand what's happening when you feel it. When you feel it, the only way to start to understand how to apply that to someone else is to get them to feel it. So it's a very strange art in that respect.

So that then raises the issue of how do you promote Systema in today's Youtube world?

It is a difficult thing to promote, but I think you do it through the health and fitness aspects, the well being as well as the fighting. But I guess the best way is hands-on with people, let them feel it for themselves. Those that want to do it will do it, others won't. And I'm not saying that people in Systema shouldn't do other things too. I have a school with some top guys in MMA and BJJ, it would be crazy for me to tell my students not to train with them.

How did the Academy come about? It's a great thing to have such high level teachers all in one place.

A friend of mine put me and Rigan Machado (BJJ / JJ champion) together and we decided to open a school in LA. I'd been living there for 11 years or so. We found a place in Beverly Hills – there's a lot of schools in LA but not many in Beverly Hills. It's been going well! Cezar Galvao came on board (Taekwondo champion) and then John Lewis (trainer of Chuck Lidell, BJ Penn, Tito Ortez). They are all great guys, legends. Rigan has had a 365-0 fight record! It's great to have them there. We promote

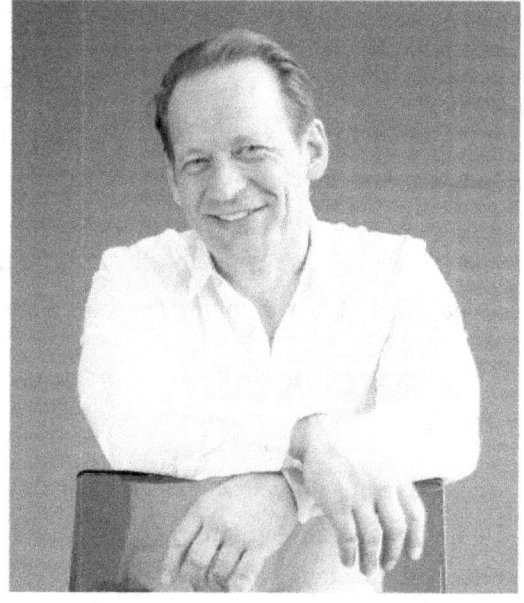

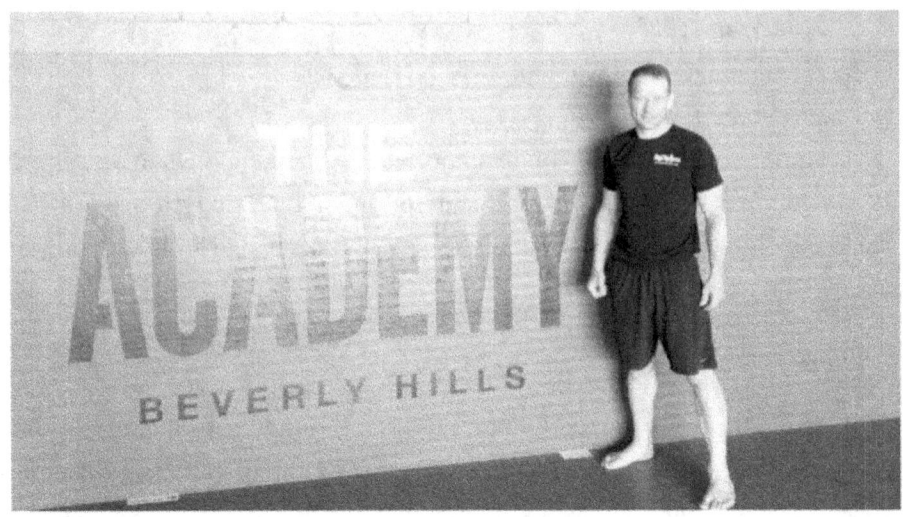

all the classes and encourage cross-training so people can see the benefits. The idea of the school was to make these high level guys accessible. It's very much about everyone helping each other to improve, being honest with your training.

I saw a photo of Dan Inosanto training in Systema recently, how did that come about?

Yes, Danny, plus Mark Denny, Jeff Imada and Mark Cheng. Danny's a black belt under Rigan. He came to say hi when we opened the school and it went from there. He's a very open guy. He told me he'd watched Systema for ten years and didn't get it, but now he's been training for a couple of years. I run an open class, he came and tried it, now he loves it. He trains with me once a week, the other guys came in through that. Jeff is one of the top Filipino guys and has done a lot of film work – The Bourne Identity, Big Trouble in Little China, Fight Club, tons of movies, he's a great guy.

Bruce Lee is the great martial arts icon. How did it feel working with people who had trained with him?

I was a huge Bruce Lee fan growing up. I was actually planning to train with Danny before coming into Systema. I went to a workshop of his back then, amazing knowledge and a great attitude. About a week after I met Vladimir and went in that direction instead. So it was great to see Danny again, he's such a humble guy, totally open. So yes, I sit there at the end of class chatting with these guys, wearing Systema t-shirts, it can feel kind of odd (laughs).

Did you ever think back in the day, on the doors at 2am in the morning, that you would ever be doing that?

That's the thing, I never really thought it wouldn't happen, but then again never thought that it would. I never really had a plan, just see how things go. I'm still that way. There's a concept in screen-writing of the diamond. The diamond shape is your life, it opens out until a certain point, where it starts closing back in. So that can make people depressed. The beautiful thing about training in something like Systema is that the diamond never turns back in. Each stage of your life is an opening to another level. It opens you up to who you are at each stage of your life. It's also one of the nice things about living somewhere like California, they don't have that age-related idea, it opens things up a lot.

Movement and exercise can be a powerful antidote to that too?

Yes, I mean look at our teachers, all in their 50s, but look at their movement. It's important also to change environments in training. Train outside, in

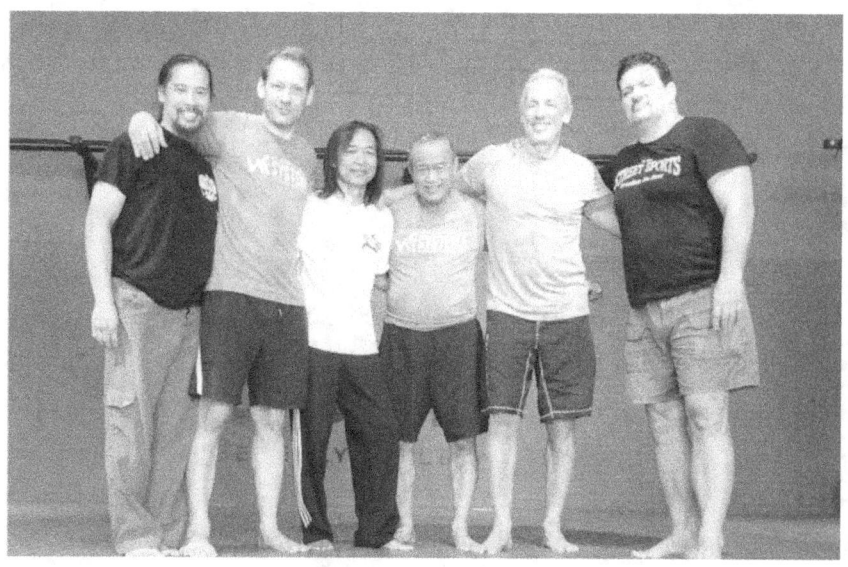

different conditions, it all helps change peoples' mindsets. Also you have to be careful in Systema not just to train with Systema people, sometimes train differently, work with different people.

When did you first train with Mikhail?

Pretty close to first starting, after about a year. He came to Toronto to do a seminar. Like everybody else, I didn't get it at first, it was hard to comprehend the things he was doing. I could feel it though (laughs). He's an incredible martial artist, unique. Someone like Mikhail hasn't been around for who knows how long – and he is here right now, you can come and train with him. It is difficult to see though – I mean if someone like Danny can't see it, how will most other people? And in some ways, if you can understand what Mikhail is doing from a video clip, he is not doing very good Systema! It's meant not to look like anything. It depends what people are looking for, same as the media, it's not what the media is looking for!

True, but if you think back to that Kung Fu series it had a strong philosophical element. I mean you knew he was going to kick ass at some point but there was that underlying calmness. Compared to now, where everyone is shouting, it's very loud and brash.

Well that's the way they have to promote MMA these days I guess. It can then become the expectation of how things are. I don't think it bothers Mikhail or Vladimir one way or the other how things are perceived. I remember when first training with Vladimir, the sheer amount of information that he was giving out – and still is. I said to him once, "You know, I've received more information here in a week than from a

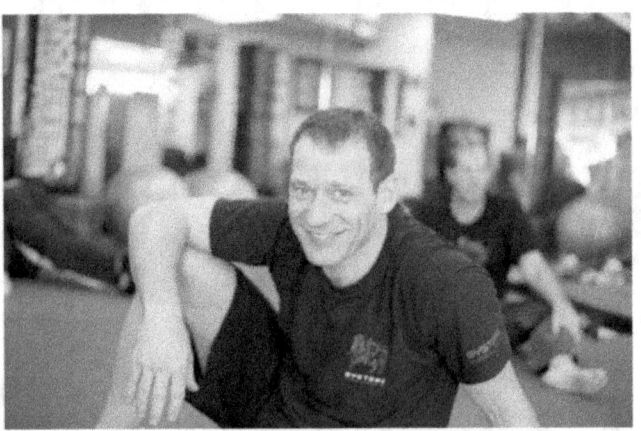

whole time training somewhere else". He said to me "Systema is a gift and should be shared". I think that's the great thing about this art, the founders are here this

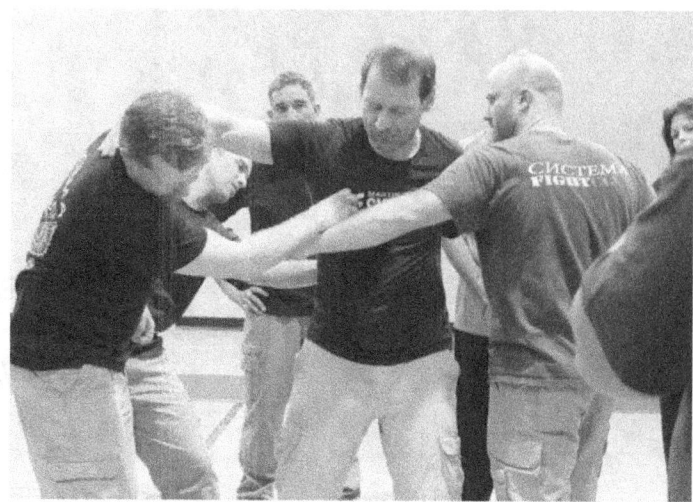

weekend, you can up to them and ask anything, go any speed you like, they are open. It means that all of us are directly under their teachings and influence. There's no egos, we are helping each other. So in that sense Systema is a slow burn.

What sorts of people come to train with you?

My students are a whole range of people, from A list actors to construction workers. People with a curious mindset are perhaps more open to Systema, they are more open to the idea of learning rather than being taught. So it's for everyone but not everyone is interested, same as not everyone is interested in MMA or whatever. It's not a concern for me in that sense, I'm more concerned with the people who are training in Systema than those who are not (laughs). What I'd say about anything is if you want to make a comment on something then try it first. The thing I hear most from the people I teach is not that I got into a fight but that I enjoy my life more. I feel more relaxed, I don't get so annoyed, I enjoy my drive to work.

You mentioned screen writing earlier, how did you get into that?

I was living in Kentucky, working as a graphic designer and always had an eye for video work and film. I was training with Vladimir at the time and thought everyone knows about Chuck Norris and those guys, but no-one knows about

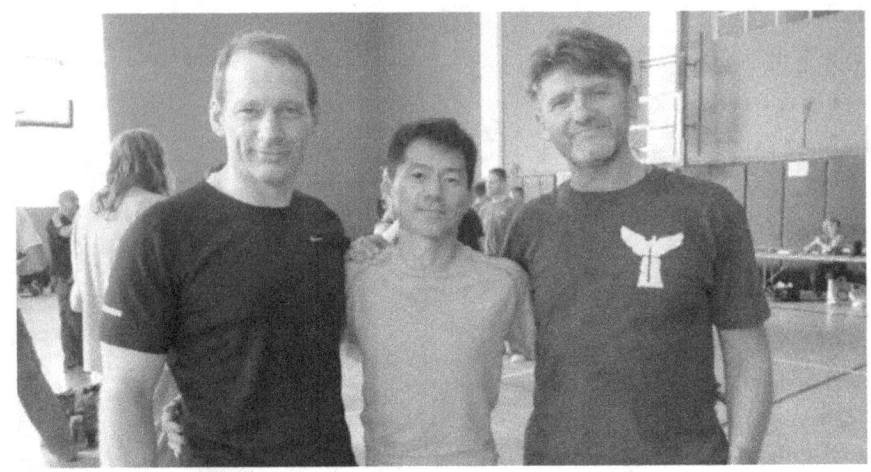

these underground guys, maybe I should do a documentary. So I got involved with a small film company in Kentucky. Nothing really came of it, but they did have some scripts which I read and thought maybe it was something I could do. I wrote a script called *Murphy's Razor* about an English cop chasing down gun runners. I just wrote it, I hadn't read any books on how to do it or anything, I just gave it a go. I had no concept of budgets or anything and thought well no-one is going to film it, so I made my own short movie.

Then it was just a weird set of circumstances. A local reporter moved in a couple of doors down to me, he heard about the film, local people had helped me make it. He loved the film and gave me a nice write up. At the time he was also working for Kate Davies, who won a Sundance award for her documentary – it later also won an Emmy. Kate loved the short too and also gave me a good write up. That should have been the end of it, no-one from Hollywood is looking for films in Kentucky!

About a week after that I got a call from LA – I didn't think it was real but I sent the film off. They got back to me and said they loved it, so I asked who they were (laughs). It turned out they were a real company. They suggested some edits, then they put the script out and it sold straight away to Gold Circle (they'd just done *My Big Fat Greek Wedding*). Russell Crowe was interested, so suddenly I had this LA career. They asked me to write another, so I locked myself away for three weeks and wrote a heist movie, *The Trouble with Stealing*. They put it out and it sold straight away, so it was obvious I had to move to LA!

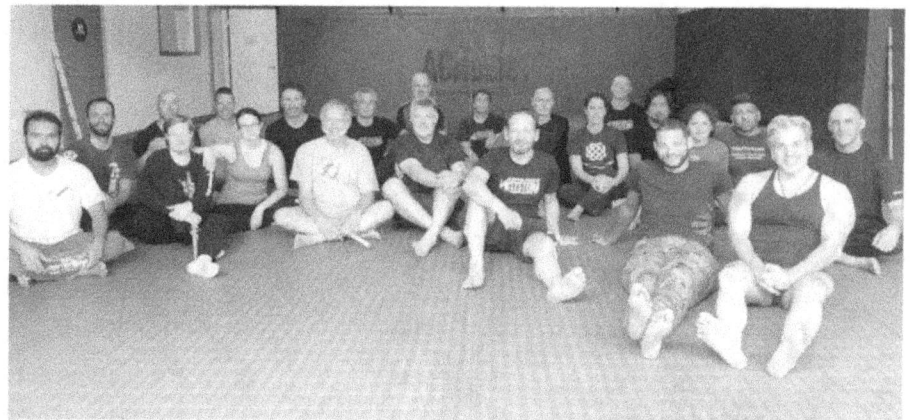

I had three studio films made in 15 months, which pushed me into the big league. I've worked with Richard Gere – he was a fun guy. I've also worked some fight choreography and worked with Wesley Snipes, he is very interested in Systema.

Do you ever see a Systema documentary being made?

I think at some point there may be. I don't think I'd be the guy to do it. But we are back to that problem – it's hard enough to understand when you are doing it, let alone watching! Maybe a film would be a more likely vehicle – there are things coming up in the future I can't really talk about, but certain people are training with us!

Speaking of film, you have some instructional titles out?

Yes the medicine ball workout and the stick fighting. I'm changing everything over to downloads so they are easy for people to get hold of.

What's your take on fitness training?

My concept of fitness changed a lot since starting Systema. There's always that concept of, if you are lifting weights to train lifting a body, then why not just lift a body! I think more in terms of health than fitness these days. To separate Systema from massage is difficult, that's obviously a huge part of it.

It's good to have a strong body but it must be healthy. If your fitness training restricts your movement, then why are you doing it? And that can be movement

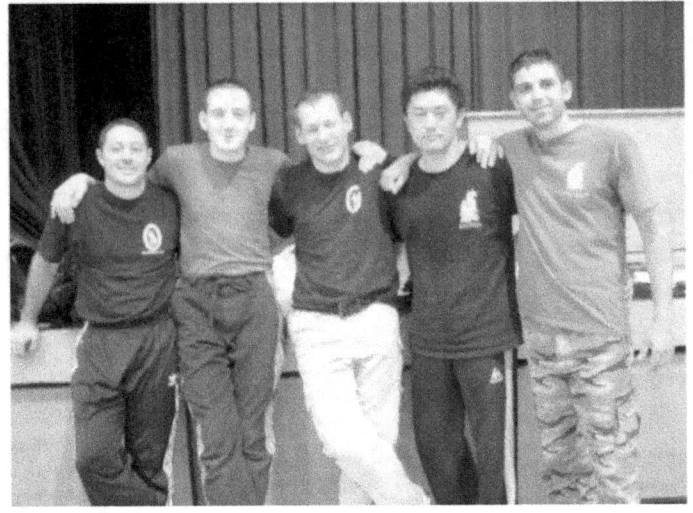

of blood, lymph, not just muscles. In the past, we'd do endless repetitions. Now I never do fitness purely for strength. If you are going to exercise you should do it only to relax, because that is true health and fitness. You die from the feet up, you get old from the feet up. I take a great joy in seeing my students shed off the years through the exercises.

Also you need to change things so you are not working one part all the time. Do push-ups to relax, squats to relax. The strength will come out of that. The best way I feel now is if I feel nothing at all. Any tension in the body is uncomfortable, it means that something is wrong. The first thing Vlad said to me was, "Don't worry about what you look like". We should work on how we feel inside, not how we look outside.

In closing do you have any thoughts about the future of Systema or what Systema means to you?

I can't say for other forms of RMA but from what I can see, Mikhail's version of Systema is very old. I've trained it a lot of arts but nothing has the depth of information. Systema has deep roots. I think it originated as a sword art, the striking and concepts are very much like a sword art, plus of course the sword was a spiritual weapon.

The hardest question I get asked is, "Systema – what is it". It's hard to explain.... Systema now means to me not trying to do some form of Systema but more trying to understand what Systema means in the sense of how I actually do things. I'm starting to understand it's more about recognising yourself. Not, "I am doing something" but more, "Who am I that is doing this" You can teach all the Systema in the world but if people don't understand the concept of a calm psyche then nothing will he happening. Or take "relax," it's a complicated terms it doesn't mean "collapse".

I remember when I first got into graphic design I learned that there's 256 levels of grey (laughs). It's the same with relaxed, there's a million gradations you have to explore and be aware of. To be relaxed is the healthiest state – no baby comes out tense. But then you get slapped! So you learn how to tense, it becomes a reaction to your environment. If you are not afraid of your environment, you have less fear and so don't tense. But you have to understand your environment for that to happen and that can be your external state and your internal state.

To me, Systema now is learning how to be a tuning fork in your environment. The Systema methodology gives you the tools you to do that.

APPENDIX ONE
CONTACT DETAILS

SYSTEMA HQ

http://systemaryabko.wixsite.com/systema

http://www.russianmartialart.com

BRAZIL

Nelson Wagner
http://www.artemarcialrussa.com.br

CANADA

Emmanuel Manolakakis
https://www.fight-club.ca

Jason Priest
http://www.russianmartialart.com

Pete Rogers
https://www.facebook.com/systemakingston

CHINA

Ali Chui
https://www.facebook.com/systemarmachin/

GERMANY

Norbert Tannert
http://systema-bonn.de

JAPAN

Ryo Onishi
http://www.systemaosaka.jp

PERU

Bratzo Barrena
http://systemarusocf.wix.com/peru

TAHITI

Jerome Laigret
http://www.systematahiti.com

UK

Matt Hill
http://www.matthill.co.uk

Robert Poyton
http://www.systemauk.com

USA

Sergey Makarenko
http://norcalsystema.com

Glen Murphy
http://www.ncsystema.com

Martin Wheeler
http://theacademybeverlyhills.com

APPENDIX TWO
FURTHER READING

Edge: Secrets of the Russian Blade Masters - Vladimir Vasiliev & Scott Meredith

Strikes - Vladimir Vasiliev & Scott Meredith

Let Every Breath - Vladimir Vasiliev

The Systema Manual - Major Konstantin Komarov

The Ten Points of Sparring - Robert Poyton

Systema Solo Training - Robert Poyton

Systema Partner Training - Robert Poyton

Systema Health - Matt Hill

Systema Combat Drills - Matt Hill

Living Systema - Matt Hill

www.ingramcontent.com/pod-product-compliance
Lightning Source LLC
Chambersburg PA
CBHW071813080526
44589CB00012B/782